中国经典谚语中的健康智慧研究

Research on the Wisdom of Health in Classical Chinese Proverbs

（汉英对照）

李晓婧　邝梦丽　张琪琪　主编

东南大学出版社
SOUTHEAST UNIVERSITY PRESS
·南京·

内 容 简 介

本书选编了中国历代典籍中及民间流传较广的健康养生谚语和格言,简单解释其意义,并将其翻译成英文。此外,每一谚语或格言下还扼要补充了与之有关的健康知识,以期在帮助读者重温、学习传统文化的同时,树立健康意识,培养良好的生活习惯,促进身心健康。

图书在版编目(CIP)数据

中国经典谚语中的健康智慧研究 / 李晓婧,邝梦丽,张琪琪主编. — 南京 : 东南大学出版社,2023.6

ISBN 978-7-5766-0469-6

Ⅰ. ①中… Ⅱ. ①李… ②邝… ③张… Ⅲ. ①中医典籍-普及读物 Ⅳ. ①R2-5

中国版本图书馆 CIP 数据核字(2022)第 231636 号

责任编辑:刘 坚(635353748@ qq.com) 责任校对:张万莹
封面设计:余武莉 责任印刷:周荣虎

中国经典谚语中的健康智慧研究

Zhongguo Jingdian Yanyu Zhong De Jiankang Zhihui Yanjiu

主 编:李晓婧 邝梦丽 张琪琪
出版发行:东南大学出版社
社 址:南京市四牌楼 2 号 邮编:210096 电话:025-83793330
网 址:http://www.seupress.com
电子邮箱:press@ seupress.com
经 销:全国各地新华书店
印 刷:广东虎彩云印刷有限公司
开 本:700 mm×1000 mm 1/16
印 张:12.25
字 数:240 千字
版 次:2023 年 6 月第 1 版
印 次:2023 年 6 月第 1 次印刷
书 号:ISBN 978-7-5766-0469-6
定 价:68.00 元

本社图书若有印装质量问题,请直接与营销部联系。电话:025-83791830

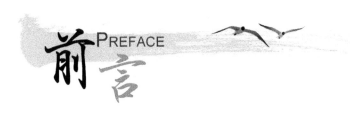

前言 Preface

　　谚语是中国古代劳动人民长期生活的经验总结,体现了中华民族的智慧与创造力。其形式言简意赅,语言通俗易懂且幽默风趣,朗朗上口,因而在大众中广为流传。谚语包罗万象,涉及面十分广泛,有的反映了气象与农业,有的则反映了劳动人民对养生保健、延年益寿的积极追求。

　　谚语中的健康养生智慧,与中国传统医学有着紧密的联系,富具科学性与实用性。在收集整理的过程中,笔者发现多数健康养生谚语出自中医典籍,如《黄帝内经》中的"精神内守,病安从来"、《抱朴子》中的"忍怒以全阴气,抑喜以养阳气"等;亦有些谚语来自中国古代经典著作,如《论语》中的"食无求饱,居无求安";更有些谚语出处不详,通过人们口口相传而流传至今,如"心胸宽大能撑船,健康长寿过百年"。

　　近几年来,受疫情的影响,人们强烈感受到了中医药的奥秘与功用,对健康养生的需求也越来越迫切。本书从上述来源中选取了两百余条经典的有关健康的谚语,并将其划分为情志、饮食、运动、季节四大篇,不仅阐释了其中的养生哲理,且提供了可供参考的健康小提示,对于现代人们了解养生常识、祛病延年不无裨益。

　　鉴于中国传统医药文化在国际上影响力的日趋增强,本书特意编排为汉英双语版,希望能够为外语读者提供些许帮助,但中国经典谚语广博精深,有些还有待科学考证,加之笔者的能力有限,因而语言上难免有疏漏之处,诚挚希望有关专家学者以及广大读者能够不吝赐教。

　　本书为李晓婧老师的 2022 年教育部产学合作协同育人项目"高等中医药院校中医翻译教育师资培训项目"(220901549214657)的部分成果。

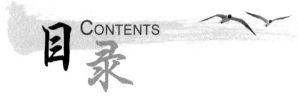

CONTENTS

目录

参考书目

附录

第一章　健康谚语情志篇
Chapter One　Health-preserving Proverbs About Emotion

第一节　精神内守
Section One　Keeping *Jingshen*（Essence and Spirit）in Interior

1 得神者昌,失神者亡。

Loss of *shen*（spirit）will cause death while maintenance of *shen*（spirit）will ensure life.

《黄帝内经》中说:"得神者昌,失神者亡。"前者指的是若病人看起来神采飞扬、精神抖擞,则说明预后良好,疾病可愈;相反,后者指的是若病人神色恍惚、精神欠佳,则说明其预后不良,疾病难愈。此句说明神对人体生命活动意义重大。在中医上,通过望神可以知虚实、测预后、决生死。

There is a saying in *Huang Di Nei Jing*（*Huangdi's Canon of Medicine*）that "Loss of *shen*（spirit）will cause death while maintenance of *shen*（spirit）will ensure life. " The former means a patient has recovered well if he/she is in high spirits after treatment; on the contrary, the patient might not recover well and the illness might be incurable if he/she is in low spirits after treatment. This shows that *shen*（spirit）is of great significance to the life activities of human body. According to traditional Chinese medicine（TCM for short）, through observing one's face,

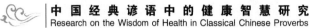
the doctors can know one's deficiency and excess, predict the effect of his/her recovery, and determine his/her life and death.

------ 健康小提示 -- Health-preserving Tips

人体养神有多种方法,最常见的莫过于闭目养神。养神的关键在于七情适度,即喜、怒、忧、思、悲、恐、惊,各有法度,适可而止。中医上讲思虑是神的一种功能,少思则神和,多思则神伤。因此,省思少虑亦是健康之道。

There are various methods to preserve one's *shen* (spirit), among which closing eyes to refresh spirit is the most common one. The key to nourishing one's *shen* (spirit) lies in the moderation of seven emotions, namely, joy, rage, worry, pensiveness, grief, terror, and fright, all of which move based on one's own natural laws. According to TCM, pensiveness is a function of *shen* (spirit). Less pensiveness is harmonious, but over pensiveness is dangerous. Therefore, keeping pensiveness in moderation is the way to preserve one's health.

2　静则神藏,躁则消亡。

If [*qi* in human body] is kept calm, *shen* (spirit) will be stored; if it is agitated, *shen* (spirit) will be exhausted.

《黄帝内经》中说:"静则神藏,躁则消亡。"五脏之气,安静则精神内守,躁动则易于耗散。中医认为,精、气、神是人体三宝,而神居首位。人体神气宜静不宜躁,因此静心可谓养神一大关键。

A saying in *Huang Di Nei Jing* (*Huangdi's Canon of Medicine*) goes that "If [*qi* in human body] is kept calm, *shen* (spirit) will be stored; if it is agitated, *shen* (spirit) will be exhausted." For *qi* in five *zang* viscera, if it is kept calm inside, *jingshen* (essence and spirit) will be stored in the interior of human body. However, if it is restless, *jingshen* (essence and spirit) will be prone to exhaust. TCM holds that the three treasures of human body are *jing* (essence), *qi* and *shen* (spirit), of which *shen* (spirit) is the first. What is better for *shen* (spirit) in human body is not restlessness but calmness, so calmness is one of the keys to nourishing the *shen* (spirit).

----- 健康小提示 ----------------------------------- **Health-preserving Tips**

如今,人们的生活及工作节奏较快,养神更显关键。养神并不难,比如下班后,回到家里洗个热水澡,或者泡泡脚,然后休息一下。这是一个保健妙招。

In modern society, the pace of one's life and work is hectic, so it is more important to nourish the *shen* (spirit). In fact, it is not difficult for one to nourish his/her *shen* (spirit). For example, after one day's work, one can take a hot bath or soak his/her feet, and then have a rest. That is a good idea to preserve his/her health.

3　多思则神殆,多念则志散,多欲则损智,多事则形疲。

Over pensiveness consumes one's heart spirit, over thought dissipates one's mind, more desires damage one's brain, and more matters lead to physical fatigue.

《养性延命录》中说:"多思则神殆,多念则志散,多欲则损智,多事则形疲。"日常生活中,人一旦思虑过多就会损耗心神,念头多了就会意志消散,欲望多了头脑便会神志不清,事情多了身体便会疲惫。因而,中医认为少思、少念、少欲、少事便是健康之法。

A saying in *Yang Xing Yan Ming Lu* (*A Collection of Health Preservation*) goes that over pensiveness consumes one's heart spirit, over thought dissipates one's mind, more desires damage one's brain, and more matters lead to physical fatigue. In daily life, one will lose his/her heart spirit because of excessive thought, dissipate his/her mind because of over intentions, become confused because of more desires, and become exhausted if one is busy with too many things. Therefore, TCM holds that less pensiveness, less thought, less desires, and less matters can promote health preservation.

----- 健康小提示 ----------------------------------- **Health-preserving Tips**

修身养性的最佳方法是少思寡欲。生活中,人们要学会调节自身的情绪和

心理状态。想问题、做事情都应在自我能力承受的范围内。身心感到疲惫时，可以通过自己喜欢的方式，比如听音乐或看剧来放松一下。

The best way for self-cultivation is to moderate our desires and thinking. In daily life, one should learn to adjust his/her own emotion and psychological state. Thinking and doing things shall be controlled within the scope of one's own capacity. When one feels tired physically or mentally, he/she can take a short break in some way, such as listening to music, watching films and TV series.

4　惜气存精更养神，少思寡欲勿劳心。

Cherishing *qi* and storing *jing*（essence）to nourish *shen*（spirit）; reducing pensiveness and desires to relax heart.

明代御医龚廷贤曾言："惜气存精更养神，少思寡欲勿劳心。"中医认为精气是构成并维持人体生命活动的基本物质之一，因此人们应惜气存精以养其内外精神。那么该如何保养精、气、神呢？其一在于少思虑；其二在于克制自身对名利和性的贪欲；其三在于动脑筋、费心思要坚持适度原则。

Gong Tingxian, imperial physician in the Ming Dynasty said that "Cherishing *qi* and storing *jing*（essence）to nourish *shen*（spirit）; reducing pensiveness and desires to relax heart." TCM believes that essential *qi* is one of the basic substances to constitute and maintain the life activities of human body. Therefore, one should cherish the essential *qi* to nourish his/her internal and external spirit. In what way one can maintain *jing*（essence）, *qi* and *shen*（spirit）? The first is to reduce pensiveness, the second is to restrain the greed for fame, gain and sex, and the last is to adhere to the principle of moderation when thinking.

------ 健康小提示 --------------------------------- **Health-preserving Tips**

中医上常说精、气、神是人体三宝。精力充沛、气血充足、神色充盈可以用来说明一个人的身心健康。闲暇时间，打打坐，练练气功，或者打打太极拳和八段锦，可以存养气血，减少繁重的思虑，达到静心养神的目的。

According to TCM, *jing*（essence）, *qi* and *shen*（spirit）are the three treasures of human body. If one is energetic, full of *qi* and blood, and has a good spirit, he can be regard as a healthy person physically and mentally. In one's free time, sitting in meditation, or doing *qigong*, *taijiquan* and *baduanjin* (eight-sectioned exercise) can nourish *qi* and blood and reduce pensiveness so as to achieve the purpose of meditation and restfulness.

5　精神内守，病安从来。

Jingshen (essence and spirit) is kept inside, and diseases will have no way to develop.

《黄帝内经》中说："精神内守，病安从来。"意思是说人的精神若内守于心而不过分消耗以致损伤，那么疾病又从何而来呢？现代医学研究发现，一切对人体有不利影响的因素中，最能使人短命夭亡的就是不良情绪。因此，保养精神在人的一生当中是至关重要的。

There is a sentence in *Huang Di Nei Jing* (*Huangdi's Canon of Medicine*) that states, "*Jingshen* (essence and spirit) is kept inside, and diseases will have no way to develop." It means that if the human spirit stored in the heart is not overly consumed or damaged, then where does disease come from? Modern medical research has found that among all the factors that are harmful to human body, the most critical one is bad emotion. Thus, preserving *jingshen* (essence and spirit) is vital to one's life.

----- 健康小提示 ----------------------------- **Health-preserving Tips**

生活中要时常保持精神愉快，心胸宽广，情绪稳定。工作和学习之余，可寻找舒适之处让身心恢复到宁静、清醒的状态当中。若遇到不顺心的事，可通过中医上的"以情制情"之法来疏解情绪。

In daily life, one shall always keep his/her spirit cheerful, his/her mind open, and his/her emotion calm. After work and study, one can find a comfortable place to restore his/her body and mind to a state of peace and sobriety. If encountering something uncomfortable, one can use the method of reconciling one bad emotion through another emotion to relieve oneself.

6 心大则百物皆通，心小则百物皆病。

If one is broad-minded, he/she will not haggle over everything; if one is narrow-minded, he/she will get ill by everything.

宋代理学家、思想家朱熹在《近思录》中曾云："心大则百物皆通，心小则百物皆病。"一个人若心胸宽广，为人谦虚豁达，那么万事万物都不会阻碍其本心；而一个人若心胸狭隘，为人斤斤计较，那么看任何事情，无论大小，都会各种挑剔，内心憋屈，久憋成病。

Zhu Xi, a thinker in the Song Dynasty, said in *Jin Si Lu* (*Reflections on Things at Hand*) : "If one is broad-minded, he/she will not haggle over everything; if one is narrow-minded, he/she will get ill by everything. " If one is broad-minded and humble, then everything will not get stuck in his/her mind; but if one is narrow-minded, he/she will be picky about everything, no matter how big or small. In the end, he/she will suffer from diseases because of long-term dissatisfaction.

------ **健康小提示** ----------------------------- **Health-preserving Tips**

日常生活中，要学会以平常心看待万事万物。遇到不顺心的事，多和家人或朋友沟通，寻找合适的排解方式。

In daily life, one should learn to look at everything with a normal mind. When something is not going well, one might communicate with families or friends to find a right way to deal with it.

7 心乱则百病生，心静则万病患。

If the heart is disordered, various diseases will arise; if the heart is calm, various diseases will be curable.

神医扁鹊曾言："心乱则百病生，心静则万病患。"人的内心平静，疾病就能治愈。而人的内心杂乱丛生，身体就会患上各种疾病。这也说明心静是保持健康的首要法则。

Bian Que, a famous ancient Chinese physician in the Spring and Autumn

Period said, "If the heart is disordered, various diseases will arise; if the heart is calm, various diseases will be curable." When one's heart remains clam, he/she will keep away from diseases, otherwise, he/she will suffer from various diseases. This also shows that keeping internal peace is the first law of health-preservation.

----- **健康小提示** ----------------------------------- **Health-preserving Tips**

中医认为人体气机与自身的情志状况密切相关,不能太过耗费心神,遇事也不要过多忧虑,不要大喜大悲。

TCM holds that the *qi* movement of human body is closely related to one's emotional state. Therefore, one should not dissipate his/her heart spirit excessively. When encountering something, one should not worry too much or be overjoyed or sad.

8　不气不愁,活到白头。

Keep away from anger and worry, and one'll live until his/her hair turns grey.

民谚"不气不愁,活到白头"旨在告诉人们不生气、不发愁有利于身心健康,长寿保命。气和愁皆是对人体健康不利的不良情绪。中医认为人体五脏气机融为一体,暴怒伤肝,殃及全身。

The proverb "Keep away from anger and worry, and one'll live until his/her hair turns grey" tells people that it is beneficial for physical and mental health to be free of anger and worry. Anger and worry are bad emotions that are not good for human health. TCM holds that the five *zang* viscera of human body are an organic whole. Great or violent anger will injure the liver, and then affect the whole body.

----- **健康小提示** ----------------------------------- **Health-preserving Tips**

缓解不良情绪,可以采用头部按摩法和足部按摩法。用双手大拇指的指腹按压两翼的太阳穴,能够有效疏解心中烦闷和身体疲劳。相对地,用食指或大拇指的指腹用力按压太冲穴(位于足部背面第一脚趾和第二脚趾趾骨之间的凹陷最深处),感到微麻为佳。

Methods of head massage and foot massage can be adopted to relieve bad emotions. Pressing Point *Taiyang* on both sides by thumbs of both hands can effectively relieve the boredom and physical fatigue. In contrast, Point *Taichong* (LR 3) should be pressed by index fingers or thumbs until one feels slight numb. [Point *Taichong* (LR 3): located in the deepest part of the depression between the first toe and the second toe on the back of the foot]

9 千保健，万保健，心态平衡是关键。

No matter how to keep healthy, psychological balance is the key.

心理平衡是保证身体健康的关键。中医认为人的情志活动与内脏有着密切的关系，如喜伤心、怒伤肝、思伤脾、悲伤肺、恐伤肾。此外，有研究表明：长期的忧虑、恐惧、愤怒会导致血压的持续升高。

Psychological balance is the key to ensuring physical health. According to TCM, human emotional activities are closely related to internal zang-organs. For example, over joy hurts the heart, over rage hurts the liver, over pensiveness hurts the spleen, over grief hurts the lung and over fear hurts the kidney. In addition, studies have shown that long-term worry, fright, and rage will cause a continuous increase in blood pressure.

------ 健康小提示 ----------------------------- **Health-preserving Tips**

在生活、工作或学习当中要学会自我暗示，调整心态，及时放松自己。平时可以多和朋友、家人参加户外活动，享受大自然，让内心静下来。

One needs to learn to self-suggest in life, work or study, adjust mentality, and relax in time. To take part in more outdoor activities with friends and families, enjoy the nature and calm down is good for keeping healthy.

10　药补不如食补，食补不如神补。

If one is broad-minded enough, he will be healthy and long-lived for a

Preserving health through diet is better than that through drugs; while preserving health through *shen*-cultivation is better than that through diet.

通过药物来补养身体，不如多吃五谷杂粮；而吃五谷杂粮，不如保养精神。现代人们的生活水平普遍提高，保健药物和各种各样的美味数不胜数，但要更注重从根源上，也即从精神上来保养身体。

Compared to drugs, food is better to preserve health. While, the best way to nourishing human body is to cultivate *jingshen* (essence and spirit). In modern society, the living standards of ordinary people have generally been improved, and there are countless health-care drugs and various delicacies. However, one should focus more on life-cultivation from the ultimate source of health, namely, spirit.

----- 健康小提示 ----------------------------- **Health-preserving Tips**

战国时期著名哲学家庄子在其所著《庄子》中最早提及养生一说。养生应当顺应自然，不被内在的情感所束缚，只有从精神上与自然界天人合一，才能够保养生命，以达长寿。

Zhuangzi, a famous philosopher in the Warring States Period firstly mentioned health preservation in his book *Zhuangzi* that health preservation should conform to nature, not be bound by inner emotions. Only harmony between man and nature is achieved, one's life can be maintained to achieve longevity.

11　心胸宽大能撑船，健康长寿过百年。

If one is broad-minded enough, he will be healthy and long-lived for a hundred years.

我国民间有"宰相肚里能撑船"的说法，与此句谚语异曲同工。心胸坦荡，有包容心，懂得宽以待人的人才能够健康长寿。中医认为心宽则百病去，健康长寿的根本在于心理健康。

There is a saying that "A great man forgives and forgets", which is similar to this proverb. Those who are broad-minded toward others can live longer and own healthy life. According to TCM, a broad mind will eliminate all diseases, and the foundation of longevity lies in mental health.

------ 健康小提示 ------------------------------- **Health-preserving Tips**

中医认为,通过饮食可以调节人的心理情绪。生活中可以适当多吃一些疏肝理气的食物,比如萝卜、芹菜、橙子、柚子等。

TCM believes that people's emotions can be regulated through diet. In daily life, one can eat more food to soothe the liver and regulate *qi*, such as carrots, celery, oranges, and grapefruit.

12 无事时不教心空,有事时不教心乱。

One should not be faineant when nothing troubles; one should not be discomposed when something occurs.

《少年进德录》中说:"无事时不教心空,有事时不教心乱。"即是说,没有事时不要让心生懒散,而有事时也不要心中慌乱。在中医上,保持心绪平稳对维持人体健康极为重要。心若因外部因素而跌宕起伏,则极易消弭人的精神,导致气郁不振,进而招致疾病。

A saying in *Shao Nian Jin De Lu* (*Records of Cultivating Virtues*) goes that "One should not be faineant when nothing troubles; one should not be discomposed when something occurs." That is to say, don't let one's mind be lazy when he/she is free, and don't get panic when something occurs. According to TCM, keeping the mood stable is extremely important for maintaining human health. If the heart is in ups and downs due to external factors, it will easily deplete one's spirit, lead to depression of *qi*, and cause diseases.

------ 健康小提示 ------------------------------- **Health-preserving Tips**

无论何时,勿忘初心,不混沌、不颓丧,为实现目标而不断努力。

At any time, one should not forget his/her original aspiration, stay away from chaos and decadence, and work hard to achieve his/her goals.

13　肝火盛，不长命。

Exuberant liver fire shortens [one's] life span.

中医学运用"取象比类"的方法，把肝比作"将军之官"，意为其秉性刚烈，有统兵御敌之威。因而，"肝火盛"习惯上成了"大怒"的代称。怒则伤肝，影响人的寿命，故曰"不长命"。

TCM holds the method of classification according to manifestation, regarding the liver as a "general officer", which means that it has the character of staunch and can lead troops to fight like a general. Therefore, "exuberant liver fire" has become a synonym for over rage. Rage hurts the liver and affects one's life span, so that is called "short life span".

------- 健康小提示 --------------------------- **Health-preserving Tips**

饮食与养肝密不可分。平时可以多吃瘦肉、鱼类、牛奶等富含蛋白质的食物，不仅可以保持肝脏所需的营养，而且能够减少有毒物质对肝脏的损害。

Diet is closely related to liver-nourishment. One can enjoy more protein-rich foods, such as lean meat, fish, milk, which can not only maintain the nutrients necessary to the liver, but also reduce the damage to the liver caused by toxic substances.

14　心怀坦荡，福高寿长。

Being broad-minded and living longer.

心怀坦荡其实就是指人对一切事物的忍耐力和宽容度。心态宽容，就能够理性看待异于自己的人和事，坦然面对人生中遇到的种种困难，有助于养成正面情绪，消除负面情绪，促进心理健康。

In fact, being broad-minded refers to one's patience and tolerance for everything. With a tolerant heart, one can be rational to treat people and things that are different from himself/herself, and can be calm to face the difficulties encountered in life, which helps one to develop positive emotions, eliminate negative emotions, and promote mental health.

----- **健康小提示** ------------------------------ **Health-preserving Tips**

多同心胸开阔的人来往,学习他们的处世之道,遇到事情时可与其商量。另外,常从正面的角度思考问题,将眼光放远、放长。如果感到愤懑,可以深呼吸,转移注意力。

It's better for one to meet others who are broad-minded, and learn norms of human behaviors from them. If encountering difficulties, one can consult with them. In addition, one should think from a positive and long-term perspective. When feeling angry, one can take a deep breath to divert one's attention.

15　要活好,心别小。
To be broad-minded to get longevity.

中医认为:"发怒是百病之源。"怒气上逆,气血不畅,危害身体五脏六腑。所以,古谚说"要活好,心别小",指要想活得好,心胸就不能狭窄。只有心胸开阔的人,才有可能拥有长寿。

TCM believes that "Rage is the root of various diseases". Rage drives *qi* to ascend, causes disharmony of *qi* and blood, and damages the five *zang* viscera and six *fu* viscera. Therefore, as an ancient proverb goes, "To be broad-minded to get longevity. " It means that if one wants to live well, he/she must learn to be a broad-minded person. Only those who are not narrow-minded can live longer.

----- **健康小提示** ------------------------------ **Health-preserving Tips**

中医认为人有七情:喜、怒、忧、思、悲、恐、惊,七情之间可相互制约,以保证气血正常运行。当我们发怒时,可以保持身体自然站立,多次深呼吸,并进行心理暗示,以快速平息心中怒气。

According to TCM, one has seven emotions: joy, rage, worry,

pensiveness, grief, terror, and fright. The seven emotions can restrict each other to ensure the normal circulation of *qi* and blood. When getting angry, one can keep his/her body standing naturally, take deep breaths several times, and perform psychological hints to appease his/her emotion quickly.

16　疲劳过度,百病丛生。

Excessive fatigue causes various diseases.

《防病贵早》中说:"疲劳过度,百病丛生。"因为人体在过度疲劳时,机体内的免疫细胞功能下降,适应外界环境的应变能力也显著下降,内分泌系统也处于紊乱状态。此时,容易患病。

A saying in *Fang Bing Gui Zao* (*Preventing Disease in Advance*) goes that excessive fatigue causes various diseases. Since when the human body is in the state of excessive fatigue, the function of immune cells in the body will decrease, and the strain ability to adapt to the external environment will also significantly decrease, and the endocrine system is also in a state of disorder, which makes one prone to be attacked by diseases at the moment.

------ 健康小提示 ------------------------------- **Health-preserving Tips**

疲劳分身体疲劳和心理疲劳。中医认为易疲劳乏力者身体弱,气血不足。就身体疲劳的人群而言,最重要的就是保证充足的睡眠。对心理疲劳的人群来讲,最主要的是要注意调节放松情绪,可以选择的方法有默想、听舒缓的音乐、唱歌、画画、弹琴等。

There are two kinds of fatigue: physical fatigue and mental fatigue. TCM holds that people who are easy to be fatigued are in poor health and have no sufficient *qi* and blood. For people with physical fatigue, the most important thing is to ensure adequate sleep. For people with mental fatigue, the most important thing is to regulate their mood to relax. For example, one can practice meditation, listen to soft music, sing, paint, play the piano, and so on.

17　天宽地宽,不如心宽。

The width of the sky and the earth is not as important as the breadth of the heart.

"天宽地宽,不如心宽"强调了人心宽广的重要性,说明为人处世要心胸宽广。对自己来说,心宽是豁达;对别人来说,心宽是包容。

"The width of the sky and the earth is not as important as the breadth of the heart" emphasizes the importance of having a broad mind. This shows that one should deal with others with an open mind. For oneself, being open-minded is generosity; and for others, inclusiveness.

------ 健康小提示 ------------------------------- **Health-preserving Tips**

人不是生来就拥有豁达的心性的。生活当中,要学会自我总结和反省,从每一次经历当中看到自己的不足,学着虚心接受别人的批评与建议,一步一步开阔心胸,提高自身修为。

One is not born with an open mind. In life, learn to do self-summary, find one's shortcomings from each experience, and to be humble to accept others' criticism and advice, can open one's mind step by step and get improved.

18　百病生于气。

Qi is the root of all diseases.

《黄帝内经》中说:"百病生于气。"意思是许多疾病的发生都与人体气血运行息息相关。因此,保持健康,必须注意补气。

There is a saying in *Huang Di Nei Jing*（*Huangdi's Canon of Medicine*）that *qi* is the root of all diseases. It means the occurrence of most diseases is closely related to the circulation of *qi* and blood in human body. Therefore, nourishing *qi* in one's body is good to keep healthy.

------ 健康小提示 ------------------------------- **Health-preserving Tips**

将黄芪、当归装入原料鸡的腹中,腹部朝上,摆上葱、姜,注入清汤,加入食

盐、黄酒、胡椒粉，大火蒸约 2 小时即可。本品能补全身之气，有强身健体之效。

Put *huangqi* (milkvetch root) and *danggui* (Chinese angelica) into the abdomen of chicken with the abdomen facing up, add green onions and ginger into it, pour into clear water, then add salt, Chinese rice wine and pepper powder, and perform high temperature steaming for about 2 hours. This food can nourish *qi* and build human body.

第二节 以情制情
Section Two Reconciling One Emotion Through Another Emotion

1 情极百病生，情舒百病除。

Extreme emotions cause diseases while eased emotions expel diseases.

人体情绪舒畅，身体则强健，疾病就不会入侵；反之，若出现极端情绪，百病就会侵袭人体，造成危害。中医认为人体的情绪活动会影响气血运行。正常的情志变化有助于气血平稳运行；但若是情绪过盛，气机就会不稳，气血就会失调，从而招致疾病。

If one feels at ease, he/she will own a strong body without diseases. On the contrary, one trapped in extreme emotions may easily suffer from various diseases. TCM holds that one's emotional activities will affect the circulation of *qi* and blood. Normal emotional changes are conducive to the smooth circulation of *qi* and blood. But if one's emotions have changed so much that the *qi* movement would be unstable, the *qi* and blood would be imbalanced, and one may incur diseases.

----- 健康小提示 ----------------------------- **Health-preserving Tips**

喜、怒、忧、思、悲、恐、惊，无论哪种情绪，都应该处于平和的状态，一旦出现

极端情绪,都会直接导致气机失调,气血运行不畅,损害人体五脏六腑,招致百病。因此,学会控制自己的情绪,做自己情绪的主人,是维持健康的最简便方法之一。

Various emotions such as joy, rage, worry, pensiveness, grief, terror, and fright should be in a peaceful state. Once extreme emotions appear, disturbances of *qi* movement and disorder of *qi* and blood will occur, and five *zang* viscera and six *fu* viscera of human body will be damaged, and diseases may occur. Therefore, one should learn to control the emotions. Being the master of one's own emotions is one of the easiest ways to keep healthy.

2 乐极生悲。

Over joy leads to sorrow.

该句谚语出自《史记》,意思是高兴到极点时,转而发生令人悲伤的事情。中医上讲"大喜伤心",当人们处于极度兴奋当中,血压便会急剧升高,不仅直接伤害心脏,还伤害大脑神经等组织,增加猝死的风险。

This proverb comes from *Shi Ji* (*Records of the Grand Historian*), which means that when one is extremely happy, something painful might happen instead. According to TCM, over joy hurts the heart. When one is in a state of extreme excitement, his/her blood pressure will increasingly rise, which not only directly hurts the heart, but also damages the nervous tissue and increases the risk of sudden death.

----- **健康小提示** ---------------------------- **Health-preserving Tips**

平常人,尤其是患有高血压、心脑血管疾病的人一定要学会克制自身的情绪,保持心平气和,心绪稳定。

A person, especially one who suffers from high blood pressure and cardiovascular diseases must learn to restrain his/her emotions and keep the mood stable.

3　乐以忘忧。

Being so happy as to forget worries.

《论语》中说:"乐以忘忧。"意思是由于快乐而忘记了忧愁。此句谚语意在强调笑对人体健康的促进作用。中医学认为"忧伤肺,喜胜忧",喜则全身气机通达,气血通畅。同时,纽约大学教授罗斯·柯赛尔发现笑声可以散发心中的积郁。

A saying in *Lun Yu* (*The Analects*) says, "Being so happy as to forget worries." It means that one is happy and forgets his sadness. This proverb is intended to emphasize that smile can promote human health. According to TCM, excessive worry hurts the lung, but joy dominates over worry. If one is happy, the *qi* movement of the whole body is accessible and the circulation of *qi* and blood is fluent. Meanwhile, Ross Kossel, professor of New York University, finds that laughter can eliminate depression in one's heart.

------ 健康小提示 ---------------------------- **Health-preserving Tips**

坏情绪难以避免。心情不好的时候,可以先找个地方调整一下,暗示自己要坚强,保持微笑。

Bad feelings are inevitable. When one is in a bad mood, he/she can find a place to adjust, and hint himself/herself to be strong and keep smiling.

4　恼一恼,老一老;笑一笑,少一少。

Annoyance makes people older, but smile makes people younger.

清代学术大师钱大昕在《恒言录》中说:"恼一恼,老一老;笑一笑,少一少。"恼和笑都是人的正常情绪,恼怒催人衰老,而常笑使人年轻。

Qian Daxin, one of prestigious academic masters in the Qing Dynasty, said in the book, *Heng Yan Lu* (*Records of Common Saying*), that annoyance makes people older, but smile makes people younger. Annoyance and smile are one's normal emotions. The former makes one older, and the latter makes one younger.

生活中可以通过加强运动和体育锻炼来改善自身的情绪,同时还可以对自己的头部、足部、四肢、背部进行按摩,以疏通经络、调节气血。

In daily life, one can adjust his/her emotions by some physical exercise. At the same time, doing massage for head, feet, limbs, and back can dredge the meridians and regulate *qi* and blood.

5 愁最伤人,忧易致疾。

Worry hurts people extremely and causes diseases easily.

清代小说作家蔡东藩在《前汉演义》中说:"愁最伤人,忧易致疾。"指的是忧愁过度会引发疾病,损伤人的身心。中医学认为思虑过度则伤脾,忧愁不解则伤肺。忧愁对人的精神伤害最大,极易致病。

Cai Dongfan, a novelist in the Qing Dynasty, said in the book, *Qian Han Yan Yi* (*The Romance in the Early Han Dynasty*), "Worry hurts people extremely and causes diseases easily." It means that excessive worry will cause diseases and damage one's mind and body. According to TCM, over pensiveness will injure the spleen, and continuous worries will injure the lung. Worry is the most harmful to one's spirit, and is prone to cause diseases.

无论是生活、工作还是学习,遇到不顺心的事,要和自己的家人或朋友多谈心,这样既能够亲近彼此,又能够释放压力,排解愁思,条畅情志。

No matter in life, work or study, when something goes wrong, one can have a chat with his/her families or friends, so that one can get close to each other, relieve stress and worry, and smooth emotion.

6　哭一哭，解千愁。

A good cry relieves a thousand worries.

中医学认为，"郁则发之"。排解不良情绪最简单的方法就是使之发泄。哭泣不但可以宽胸理气，使郁闷消除，而且还可以把压抑在体内的感情都发泄出来。但这里的哭不是说一不顺心就哭泣，而是在委屈和压力难以承受时放声大哭，有助于身体和心理健康。

TCM holds that the depression should be diffused. The easiest way to relieve bad emotions is to disperse them. Good crying can not only soothe the chest and regulate *qi*, but also relieve depression, disperse all the depressed feelings in the body. The proverb means that when one cannot bear the stress, crying is favorable to his/her physical and mental health. But it is unwise to cry when trivial matters occur.

------ 健康小提示 -- **Health-preserving Tips**

哭是个体发泄情绪的直接方式。但如果一遇到不顺心的事情就哭，反而会加重不良情绪。这里的哭指的是在情绪达到一定程度后想哭的时候不压抑心中的情绪。

Crying is a direct way for people to disperse their emotions. However, if one cries every time when something goes wrong, it will aggravate the bad emotion. Crying here refers that one won't suppress his/her emotion when it accumulates to a higher degree.

7　忍怒以全阴气，抑喜以养阳气。

Controlling one's rage to nourish *yin qi*; while controlling one's great joy to nourish *yang qi*.

《抱朴子》中说："忍怒以全阴气，抑喜以养阳气。"中医认为，人体分阴阳，大怒大喜都会使阴阳不和，故主张忍怒抑喜以平衡阴阳。该句谚语意指忍耐愤怒之情以不损害阴气，抑制喜悦之意以涵养阳气。简单来说，即是保持阴阳平和。

There is a saying in *Bao Pu Zi* (*The Master Who Embraces Simplicity*) that goes, "Controlling one's anger to nourish *yin qi*; while controlling one's great joy to nourish *yang qi*." TCM believes that human body is divided into *yin* and *yang*. Rage and great joy will cause the disharmony of *yin* and *yang*. Therefore, it is advocated to control rage and great joy to balance *yin* and *yang*. This proverb focuses the importance of controling rage so as not to harm *yin qi* and restraining great joy to nourish *yang qi*. That is to keep balance between *yin* and *yang*.

------ 健康小提示 ----------------------------- **Health-preserving Tips**

养阳,最简单的方法就是多晒太阳,并且尽量选在上午阳气生发时晒太阳为宜;滋阴最好的方法就是保持心态平稳,每日睡觉前可进行几次深呼吸。

The easiest way to nourish *yang* is to bask in the sun, and it is better to do it in the morning when *yang qi* is generated. The best way to nourish *yin* is to maintain a stable mind and take several deep breaths every day before going to bed.

8　以情制情。

Reconciling one emotion through another emotion.

以情制情就是说用另一种情绪来代替或缓解当前的情绪。中医认为,怒能制忧、忧能制恐、怒能制喜、喜能制悲、悲能制怒。比如,喜则气和志达,营卫通利,百脉畅通,千愁得解。

The method of reconciling one emotion through another emotion refers to replacing or easing the current emotion by emotional changes. TCM argues that rage dominates continuous worry, worry dominates terror, terror dominates joy, joy dominates grief, and grief dominates rage. For example, when one is happy, the *qi* is harmonious, the mind is unobstructed, and all vessels are smooth, so that worries are eliminated.

------ 健康小提示 ----------------------------- **Health-preserving Tips**

以喜制悲法:当感到难过、失意的时候可以看看手边的笑话书,刷刷多媒体

搞笑小视频来转移一下自己的注意力。

The method of controlling grief by joy：When one feels sad or frustrated，he/she can read the joke book at hand or swipe the funny videos to distract his/her attention.

9　心胸坦荡荡，身体健壮壮；心情乐悠悠，身体雄赳赳。

Being broad-minded to be strong；being joyful to be energetic.

该句谚语是说宽广的胸怀可以使人身心愉悦，保持健康。中医学认为，五脏生五志，精神情志过激会引发疾病，伤及内脏，危害生命。适当的喜悦是精神安慰剂，有助于身心健康，而悲伤忧愁是精神刺激物，损害身心。

The proverb says that a broad mind can make one feel happy physically and mentally and keep healthy. Under the guidance of TCM, the five *zang* viscera produce the five minds. Extreme emotions will cause diseases, damage human organs and do harm to human life. Appropriate joy is a spiritual placebo that can help physical and mental health, while grief and worry are mental stimulants that damage human body and mind.

------ 健康小提示 ----------------------------- **Health-preserving Tips**

人要有宽广的胸怀，学会控制自己的情绪，消除恐惧、抑郁、忧虑等负面情绪，培养积极乐观、快乐向上的积极情绪。

One should build a broad mind, control his/her own emotions, eliminate negative emotions such as fear, depression, and anxiety, and cultivate positive emotions.

10　快活保寿命，气恼成了病。

Happiness contributes to health, while annoyance leads to diseases.

该句民谚意在强调情绪对健康的重要性。人心中感到快活就会产生高兴、正面的情绪，这样有利于健康长寿；而生气则会引疾病上身。中医上认为怒为肝志，怒则气逆、血堵，导致昏厥猝死。

The proverb emphasizes the importance of emotions for health preservation. If there are no worries in one's heart, he/she will feel happy, which is helpful for health and longevity. However, if one is annoyed, illness may be caused. According to TCM, the liver is associated with anger in emotion. Anger will lead to *qi* counterflow and blood blockage, resulting in fainting, or even sudden death.

----- 健康小提示 ---------------------------------- **Health-preserving Tips**

平时要修养身心,开阔心胸,通过多种途径将心中的愤懑发泄出来。可以多听一些舒缓的轻音乐来放松心灵,或者进行一些适当的运动来排解情绪。

Normally, one should cultivate his/her body, broaden his/her mind, and vent the anger in various ways. People can listen to light music to get relaxed, and take some appropriate exercise to relieve bad feelings.

11　喜伤心,怒伤肝,恐伤肾,思伤脾,忧伤肺。

[Great] joy hurts the heart, rage hurts the liver, terror hurts the kidney, pensiveness hurts the spleen, and grief hurts the lung.

《黄帝内经》中说:"喜伤心,怒伤肝,恐伤肾,思伤脾,忧伤肺。"意思是说喜、怒、恐、思、忧要适度,不要过分,过分了就有可能会危害身体。

There is a saying in *Huang Di Nei Jing* (*Huangdi's Canon of Medicine*) that goes, "[Great] joy hurts the heart, rage hurts the liver, terror hurts the kidney, pensiveness hurts the spleen, and grief hurts the lung." It implies that emotions such as joy, rage, terror, pensiveness, and worry should be moderate. Excessive emotions may harm the human body.

----- 健康小提示 ---------------------------------- **Health-preserving Tips**

要达到心平气和,五情适度,就要顺乎自然,遇事不强求,不以物喜不以己悲。

To achieve peace of mind and moderate five emotions, one must follow the laws of nature and do not insist on something extremely. One should not be pleased by external gains, or saddened by personal losses.

12　人无忧，故自寿。

One has no sorrow, and he will live longer.

宋温州人（今浙江温州）郑伯谦曾言"人无忧，故自寿"，即是说人没有忧愁烦恼，自身能够达到长寿。中医学认为忧则伤肺。人一旦心生忧愁和焦虑，就会潜移默化地影响体内正常的气血运行，导致气血紊乱，影响五脏六腑的功能，最终威胁人体健康。

Zheng Boqian was born in Wenxhou, Zhejiang province. He once said, "One has no sorrow, and he will live longer." That is to say, if one has no worries, he/she will be long-lived. TCM believes that grief hurts the lung. Once one is worried and anxious, the normal circulation of *qi* and blood in the body will be affected, the disorders of *qi* and blood may be caused, which influences the functions of five *zang* viscera and six *fu* viscera, and threatens the health in the end.

------ 健康小提示 ----------------------------- **Health-preserving Tips**

感到忧虑时，切忌一头乱麻，要先冷静分析导致忧虑的原因，进而寻找相应的解决办法，并以积极的心态去应对。

When being worried, one must not be confused. The first thing one should do is to make analysis of the worries caused, and then find the corresponding solutions to deal with it with a positive attitude.

13　善制怒，寿无数。

Being good at controlling rage contributes to longevity.

善于制止自身的怒气，才有利于健康长寿。中医认为："发怒是百病之源。"经常发怒对身心损害很大，甚至五脏六腑都会蒙受其害。这里的制怒不是说压抑怒气，而是强调自身要寻找合理的方式排解怒气以达到制止的目的。

Being good at controlling rage is conducive to health and longevity. TCM holds that Anger is the root of all diseases. Frequent anger is very harmful to the body and mind, and even damages five *zang* viscera and six *fu* viscera. The method of controlling rage does not mean repressing this emotion forcibly, but rather emphasizing the need to find reasonable ways to relieve anger so as to achieve the purpose of elimination.

情绪暴躁时,可以选择一个安静的地方放声呼喊以排解心中怨气,达到自我控制怒气的目的。

When being irritable, one can find a quiet place to shout loudly to resolve the grievances in one's heart and achieve the purpose of controlling emotions by oneself.

14 大喜荡心,微抑则定;甚怒烦性,稍忍即歇。

Great joy hurts the heart, slight restraint makes it stable; rage makes people irritable, slight tolerance makes it disappear.

《退庵随笔》有言:"大喜荡心,微抑则定;甚怒烦性,稍忍即歇。"说的是遇到令人大喜的事而心潮涌动时,略微抑制便可安定内心;遇到使人暴怒的事而性情烦躁时,稍加忍耐就可平息怒气。

Tui An Sui Bi (*Essay of Tui An*) tells people that great joy hurts the heart, slight restraint makes it stable; rage makes people irritable, slight tolerance makes it disappear. It's said that when one encounters something exciting and becomes excited, one's heart can be calm with slight restraint; when one encounters something annoying, one's anger can be eliminated with slight tolerance.

色彩在一定程度上有助于人的身体健康。闲暇时,可以多去葱郁的树林中或安静的公园里散步,昂首看蓝天白云,俯首赏百花青草,来平复心情。

Color is beneficial to human health to some extent. In the leisure time, one can go for a walk in the lush woods or quiet parks, enjoy the blue sky and white clouds and the flowers and green grass, so as to calm down.

15　大怒不怒，大喜不喜，可以养心。

When one tends to rage but not get angry，and wants to be overjoyed but not get excited，his/her heart can be nourished.

《处世悬镜》有言："大怒不怒，大喜不喜，可以养心。"本句谚语指的是当人极为恼怒时而制止怒气，保持心平气和，极为喜悦时而不得意忘形，可以修养身心。中医认为心平气和，五体方得安宁，过分极端的情绪不利于人体真气的正常运行。

As a saying in *Chu Shi Xuan Jing* (*Wisdom of Conducting Yourself*) goes, "When one tends to rage but not get angry，and wants to be overjoyed but not get excited，his/her heart can be nourished." This proverb means that when one is extremely angry or happy，he/she keeps the mind calm，his/her body and mind can be nourished. TCM believes that only if the mind is kept calm can five body constituents be peaceful. Extreme emotions are not conducive to the normal circulation of the genuine *qi* in human body.

----- 健康小提示 ----------------------------------- **Health-preserving Tips**

养心重在保持心平气和。生活当中，可以在家中练习打坐。打坐时要衣着宽松，保持身体平稳，姿势端正；要做到摒除一切杂念，只关注当下的一呼一吸，不为外界动静和自身思维所困扰。

Nourishing heart relies on mental calm. In daily life，one can practice meditation at home. When meditating，one should wear loose clothes，keep the body stable，and have a regular posture. One should get rid of all distractions，only focus on the current breath，and not be bothered by outside world and their own thinking.

第三节　怡情养性
Section Three　Contribution to Peace of Mind
and Inner Tranquility

1　精神空虚催人老,生活多彩寿缘高。

Barren spirit makes one look old, while colorful life helps one to live longer.

这句话来自民间保健谚语,含义是:若生活空虚、神无所依,人往往会加快衰老。相反,丰富多彩的生活则往往使人增加寿命。这是一种娱乐养生方式,通过多样的、积极的活动让原本枯燥的生活变得轻松愉悦,在快乐的氛围中颐养心神,调畅情志,以达到强身健体的目的。

This sentence comes from folk health-preserving proverbs, and its meaning is that one may grow old faster when his/her lives are not enriched. On the contrary, colorful life tends to increase one's life span. This is a way of health preservation through entertainment. Life can be colorful and cheerful with various and active activities. One should nourish the heart and spirit and stabilize the emotions in the atmosphere full of happiness, so as to achieve the desired effect of body building.

------ **健康小提示** --- **Health-preserving Tips**

丰富自己的生活,选择一些多样化、动静结合、刚柔相济的娱乐活动,使生活多姿多彩,既能调养身心,又能强身健体。

For enriching the life, one can choose some activities with association of activity. This can not only nourish the spirit, but also build the body.

2　业余爱好广,胜过增营养。

A wide range of hobbies are better than nutrition supplement.

有这样一条民谚:业余爱好广,胜过增营养。要知道,业余爱好不仅可以增加生活乐趣,还是一种思想营养的来源。一项业余爱好,实际上就是一个保障身体运转正常的"安全阀"。近来有诸多医学权威认为:业余爱好具有疗病强身的作用。因此,要有自己的业余爱好,这样才能有助于身体健康。

A folk proverb goes that "A wide range of hobbies are better than nutrition supplement." Hobbies can not only increase the joy of life, but also be a source of ideological nutrition. A hobby is actually a "safety valve" to ensure the normal operation of human body. Recently, many medical experts believe that hobbies have the effect of healing and strengthening the body. Therefore, one should have his/her own hobbies so as to contribute to health.

----- 健康小提示 ----------------------------------- **Health-preserving Tips**

积极培养属于自己的业余爱好,比如绘画、收藏等,这样既可以丰富自己的生活,又有利于身心健康。

One should actively cultivate his/her own hobbies, such as painting and collecting. This will not only enrich one's life, but also benefit one's physical and mental health.

3　饭养人,歌养心。
Food cultivates human body and song nourishes human spirit.

"饭养人,歌养心"是老百姓耳熟能详的一句健康谚语,它的意思是说,饭食能够保养身体,而唱歌则能修养心灵。中医学上认为,一方面唱歌能锻炼心肺功能,经常唱歌的人大多会有一个好心情。另一方面,唱歌促进人体情感的宣泄,释放郁气。所以,唱歌有促进全身气血流通的作用。

"Food cultivates human body and song nourishes human spirit" is a well-known proverb about health. It means that food has the effect of maintaining the body, while singing has the effect of cultivating the spirit. TCM holds that on the one hand, singing improves the cardiopulmonary function; on the other hand, it contributes to emotional release. One who sings often has a good mood. Therefore, singing has the effect of promoting the circulation of *qi* and blood of the whole body.

一些医学专家指出,唱歌和练气功相似,都需要端正姿势,高度集中精神,采用腹式呼吸,屏除杂念。既然唱歌如同在练气功,它能够宣泄郁结之气就理所当然了。

Some medical experts point out that singing is similar to *qigong*. Both of them require correct posture, high concentration, abdominal breathing, and elimination of distractions. Therefore, it is natural that singing can dissipate the stagnant *qi*.

4 常在花间走,活到九十九。
Often walking among the flowers and living to be ninety-nine.

民间流传着"常在花间走,活到九十九"的说法。对老人而言,收到鲜花不如徜徉在花海,不仅浪漫,还有保健功效。中医认为,老人在花间行走具有香疗作用。《神农本草经》中记载了香味对濡养人体正气的作用。

There is a folk proverb that goes, "Often walking among the flowers and living to be ninety-nine." For the elderly, it is better to walk and enjoy in the sea of flowers than receiving flowers. It is not only romantic, but also contributes to health preservation. TCM believes that walking among the flowers for elderly has the effect of aromatherapy. The book, *Shen Nong Ben Cao Jing* (*Herbal Classic of Shen Nong*) records the effect of fragrance for nourishing the healthy *qi* in human body. The scent of flowers can make the elderly relaxed physically and mentally, which has the effect of prevention as well as cure of diseases.

老年人每天可以打理打理花草,移盆、换盆、松土、施肥、浇水、剪枝等。如此可调动全身多处肌肉,锻炼身体。

The elderly can water flowers and plants every day, perform tasks such as moving pots, changing pots, loosening soil, fertilizing, watering, and pruning. By doing so, the muscles can be mobilized, and the body can be built.

5　打拳练身，打坐养性。

Doing *taijiquan* builds the body; sitting in meditation cultivates the temperament.

打拳有助于强身健体，打坐有助于调养心性。此句谚语是在强调动静结合以达健康。打拳属动，打坐属静。适当的运动能锻炼身体。打坐能让你更好地控制自己的情绪，减轻压力。动静都对健康有益。

Doing *taijiquan* helps to strengthen the body and sitting in meditation helps to regulate and nourish the temperament. This proverb emphasizes health preservation should be performed with association of activity and inertia. *Taijiquan* is dynamic, while meditation is static. Appropriate exercise makes one's body strong. Meditation will help one control his/her emotions and reduce stress. Both dynamic and static exercise is good for health.

------ 健康小提示 ---------------------------- **Health-preserving Tips**

每天保持打坐的良好习惯，有助于涵养性情，延年益寿。此外，打太极拳时要心平气和，不想不做与打拳无关的事。

Keeping meditation every day is helpful to cultivate temperament and prolong life. In addition, one should be calm, not think, and not say anything unrelated to *taijiquan* when he/she does it.

6　养心莫若寡欲，至乐无如读书。

Nothing is better than reducing desires to nourish heart; nothing is better than reading to get joy.

民族英雄郑成功曾言："养心莫若寡欲，至乐无如读书。"意思是没有比抑制贪欲更有益于身心的，没有比读书更令人快乐的。读书不仅能开拓知识，启迪智慧，还具有娱乐、调心和养生的作用。

Zheng Chenggong, a national hero, once said, "Nothing is better than reducing desires to nourish heart; nothing is better than reading to get joy. " It implies that reducing greed is better for physical and mental health than anything else, and nothing is more enjoyable than reading. Reading can not only develop knowledge and enlighten wisdom, but also play a role in entertainment, mental activity regulation and health preservation.

----- **健康小提示** ------------------------------- **Health-preserving Tips**

读书对人的精神和身体都有很大影响,能够起到修身养性的作用,在读书时可以定时闭目休息或者是做眼保健操,按摩能够促进眼部的血液循环,减少眼部疲劳。

Reading has a great impact on one's mind and body, and plays a role in self-cultivation. When reading, one can regularly close his/her eyes to rest or perform eye exercises. Massage can promote eye blood circulation and reduce eye fatigue.

7 娱乐养生,逆乐害生。

[Moderate] entertainment is good for health-preservation, but indulgence is bad for it.

该句谚语说明了娱乐与人体健康之间的关系。正常适度的娱乐有益于养心养神,而若沉迷于娱乐,难以自拔,就会极大消耗心神,大伤元气,久而久之,疾病上身。

This proverb explains the relationship between entertainment and human health. Normal and moderate entertainment is conducive to nourishing the heart and spirit, but if one indulges in it, his/her mind and original *qi* will be damaged greatly, which may induce diseases in the long run.

----- **健康小提示** ------------------------------- **Health-preserving Tips**

娱乐要注意因人而异,量力而行。

Recreational activities should vary with each individual, according to one's ability.

8　勤于书画,益寿延年。

Being diligent in calligraphy and painting promotes longevity.

谚语"勤于书画,益寿延年"意思是说经常练习写字、作画有助于培养人的心性,促进身体健康,达到益寿延年的目的。中医认为书画具有涵养健康之功效,当挥笔时,全身之气凝于手中,不仅活动了关节,而且锻炼了头脑。

The proverb "Being diligent in calligraphy and paintings promotes longevity" means that frequent practice of handwriting and painting can help cultivate one's mind, promote his/her physical health, and gain the longevity. TCM holds that calligraphy and painting have health-preserving function. When the brush is swiped, the body's energy is condensed in the hand, which not only moves the joints, but also trains the brain.

----- **健康小提示** ------------------------------ **Health-preserving Tips**

练习书法和绘画时,一定要注意自己的姿势。头要正,身要直,肩要松。

When practicing calligraphy and painting, one should pay attention to his/her posture, that is, keep his/her head and body straight, and shoulders loose.

9　常把舞来跳,痴呆不会到。

Dancing often can prevent dementia.

舞蹈能够娱乐身心,活动筋骨,是保健妙招之一。经常跳舞能够增加人体的肺活量,增强心肺功能,所以对预防慢性心血管疾病有好处。

Dancing can entertain the body and mind and move the muscles and bones. So it is a great choice for health preservation. Regular dancing can enhance one's vital capacity and cardiopulmonary function, so it is good for the prevention of chronic cardiovascular diseases.

----- **健康小提示** ------------------------------ **Health-preserving Tips**

跳舞时要注意预防受伤,提前做伸腿拉筋等热身运动,避免突然的运动对身

体造成损伤。选用的舞蹈场地要宽敞通风。

One should be careful not to get injured while dancing, and do warm-up exercises such as leg stretching in advance to avoid the damage because of sudden movements. The chosen dance venue should be spacious and ventilated.

10 跳绳踢毽,病少一半。

Skipping rope and kicking shuttlecock greatly improve patients' conditions.

跳绳、踢毽子是我国传统娱乐游戏,可以视为轻运动量的体育活动。跳绳对全身经络都有一定的刺激作用;经常踢毽子,既能增强肌肉、骨骼的功能,又能避免关节僵化。

Rope skipping and shuttlecock kicking are traditional games in China, which can be regarded as light sports. Rope skipping has stimulating effect on the meridians of the whole body. Regular shuttlecock kicking can not only strengthen the muscles and bones, but also avoid the stiffening of joints.

------ 健康小提示 ------------------------------ **Health-preserving Tips**

跳绳、踢毽的时候要量力而行,长期坚持。踢毽子有多种方式,可以根据兴趣和能力选择单人踢、双人踢。

One should do the exercise of skipping rope and kicking shuttlecock according to his/her own ability and stick to it for a long time. There are many ways to kick shuttlecock. One can choose single kick or double kick according to his/her interest and ability.

11 善弈者长寿。

Those who are proficient in playing [Chinese] chess may be long-lived.

棋类活动不仅能丰富人们的业余生活,调节精神,而且还能锻炼人的思维,提高智力,延缓衰老。所以,自古就有"弈者长寿"之说。下棋可以充实老人们的精神生活,在谈笑搏杀之间品味其中的乐趣。同时,下棋也是一种有益的社交活动,通过棋类活动,广交棋友,能增进友谊,消除孤独感,并使精神有所寄托。

Chess activities can not only enrich one's spare time and cultivate his/her spirit, but also exercise thinking ability, improve intelligence, and delay senescence. Therefore, since ancient times, there has been a proverb that "Those who are proficient in playing〔Chinese〕chess may be long-lived." Playing chess can enrich the cultural life of old people who can enjoy the joy during the process of talking, laughing and playing. At the same time, playing chess is also a beneficial social activity. Through chess activities, one can make friends to increase friendship among players, eliminate loneliness, and find spiritual sustenance.

----- 健康小提示 ---------------------------- **Health-preserving Tips**

老年人由于生理原因,脏腑功能日渐衰退,脑髓肾精不足,思维记忆不如从前,倘若能经常下棋,促使大脑不断运转,对延缓衰老、防止大脑功能的退化是颇为有益的。

Due to physiological reasons, for the elderly, the function of the viscera is gradually deteriorating, the brain and kidney essence are insufficient, and the thinking ability and memory are degenerating. If one can play chess regularly, the continuous use of brain is quite effective in delaying senescence and preventing the deterioration of the brain function.

12　游山玩水,益寿延年。

To enjoy the travelling, to prolong your life.

人的身体健康长寿,不过早衰老,需要有两个基本条件:一是体魄健,脏器安;二是精神爽,情志舒。在游山玩水中,可以呼吸到新鲜的空气,使人清醒头脑,还可沐浴阳光,流通气血,增进健康。对年轻人来说,有利于提高工作效率;对老年人而言,能益寿延年。

Keeping healthy and preventing pro-senescence need two basic conditions: one is strong body and healthy organs; and the other is good spirit with peaceful

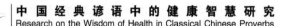
emotions. When making a sightseeing tour, one takes a fresh breath to keep a fresh mind, and enjoy the sunshine to promote the circulation of *qi* and blood so as to improve his/her own health. For the young, it is conducive to improving work efficiency; for the elderly, it can improve longevity.

----- **健康小提示** ---------------------------------- **Health-preserving Tips**

游山玩水一定要量力而行。爬山路时,保持步伐平稳、缓慢。特别是在人多路陡的地方,更要小心谨慎,防止与人碰撞或摔跤。

One should travel according to his/her physical ability. When walking along the mountain road, one should keep his/her steps slow and steady. In places of many people or steep roads, one must be careful not to push or fall.

13 常打太极拳,益寿又延年。
Doing *taijiquan* regularly contributes to prolonging one's life.

太极拳是国家级非物质文化遗产,流派众多,群众基础广泛,非常具有生命力。太极拳动作复杂,刚柔相济,绵绵不断,能很好地培养人体的协调性和平衡性。中医认为常练太极拳,可以健肾,延年益寿。

Taijiquan is the national intangible cultural heritage with many schools. It owns broad masses, and has strong vitality. The strikes of *taijiquan* are complex and combined with hardness and softness, which can well cultivate the coordination and balance of human body. TCM holds that doing *taijiquan* regularly can strengthen the kidney and prolong life.

----- **健康小提示** ---------------------------------- **Health-preserving Tips**

初学太极拳时宜慢不宜快,先把动作学会,再把要领掌握好。每次锻炼的时间长短、趟数多少、运动量大小,应根据工作和学习情况及自己的体质而定。

When learning *taijiquan*, it is better to be slow rather than fast. Learn the steps first, and then master the main points. The time and frequency of each exercise should be determined according to the work and study conditions and one's own physique.

14 早起打坐，一天快活。
Waking up early to meditate can own a nice day.

闭目盘膝而坐，调整气息出入，手放在腿上，不想任何事情。中医认为每天打坐可以矫正背部姿势，缓解脊椎压力，对于调节脊柱畸形有一定的益处。打坐可以减缓压力，帮助人体调整气血，提高抗病能力。每天打坐时间控制在半小时到一个小时。

Sit cross-legged with eyes closed, adjust the breath in and out, put hands in the lap and think about nothing. TCM believes that keeping meditation every day can correct the back posture, relieve the pressure on the spine, which is beneficial to adjust the deformity of the spine. In addition, meditation can relieve one's stress, regulate the *qi* and blood of human body, and improve the ability of disease resistance. The daily meditation time should be controlled between half an hour to an hour.

----- 健康小提示 ----------------------------- **Health-preserving Tips**

早起打坐时需要特别注意保暖。静坐时不能受"风邪"。练习者不要在寒冷的地面上打坐，不能坐在能吹到后背风的位置，静坐时不能把腰部、肚脐暴露在外面。

Keep warm when one wakes up early to meditate. Wind pathogen must be avoided during meditation. That is to say, one cannot sit on a cold ground or a place where the wind blows against his/her back. One should not expose his/her waist and belly button during meditation.

第二章　健康谚语饮食篇
Chapter Two　Health-preserving Proverbs About Diet

第一节　饮食有节
Section One　Keeping a Balanced Diet

1　饮食自倍,肠胃乃伤。
Overeating impairs the intestines and stomach.

　　《黄帝内经》中说:"饮食自倍,肠胃乃伤。"意思是说饮食过多,超过了身体所能消耗的量,就会损害肠胃。中医认为"胃为水谷之海",具有腐熟谷物,化生精微物质以供身体所需的功能,但这种功能是有限度的,因此必须根据自身身体情况合理饮食。

　　There is a saying in *Huang Di Nei Jing*(*Huangdi's Canon of Medicine*) that overeating impairs the intestines and stomach. It means that if one takes in too much food that exceeds the amount of energy consumption of his/her body, the intestines and stomach will be damaged. According to TCM, stomach is the reservoir of water and grain, which has a function of decomposing grains and producing refined nutritious substances to support human body. But this function is limited, so one's diet should be compatible with his/her physical condition.

----- 健康小提示 ----------------------------------- **Health-preserving Tips**

　　人在不同年龄阶段,脾胃的功能也会随之而变,因此,吃多吃少应根据自身

状况来调整,不可过度节食或大吃大喝。

The functions of spleen and stomach change with age. Therefore, the amount of food should be adjusted according to one's own physical condition. Excessive diet or excessive eating and drinking should be avoided.

2　要想身体好,每餐七分饱。

To be healthy, to leave off with an appetite.

民以食为天,人活着都要吃饭。俗话说得好:要想身体好,每餐七分饱。这句谚语从饮食的角度强调了保持健康的一个重要原则:食不过饱。吃得过饱,容易加重心脏负担,引发肥胖病、胃病,导致骨质疏松。

Food is the paramount necessity of the people. Everyone has to eat when he/she is alive. As the saying goes, if one wants to be in good health, he/she should eat until 70% full. From the perspective of diet, the proverb emphasizes an important principle of keeping fit: Eat not to fullness. Overeating is prone to increase the burden on the heart, cause obesity and stomach illness, and lead to osteoporosis.

----- 健康小提示 ------------------------------ Health-preserving Tips

控制用餐时间:一是按时按点吃饭,给肠胃规律的消化吸收和休息时间;二是要控制吃饭用时,以不超过 1 个小时为宜;三是要注意用餐环境;四是要合理安排用餐顺序。

The following principles are important concerning eating. Firstly, one should control the meal time: one should eat regularly and punctually so that the intestines and stomach have regular time to digest and have a rest. Secondly, one should control the time for eating, which should not exceed 1 hour. Thirdly, one should choose a comfortable place for meal. Finally, one should arrange the order of meals in a reasonable manner.

3 早食好,午食饱,晚食少。

Eating well for breakfast, eating to the full for lunch, eating less for supper.

该句谚语传达了经典的健康常识:早饭应该注重质量,午饭可以稍吃饱一些,而晚饭要稍吃少一些。一日之计在于晨,早晨是一天的开始,因此早餐要吃好一点;经过了一上午的劳动,不仅身体的能量需要补充,还要为下午的活动储备能量,因此午餐可以酌情多吃一点;而到了晚上,人基本进入休息状态,所以晚餐要相对吃少一点。

This proverb shows the classic health-preserving common knowledge: one should eat well for breakfast, eat to the full for lunch and eat less for supper. Morning is the best time of the day to work. Morning is the beginning of the day, so the breakfast should be better. After half-day's work, one should not only replenish the energy consumed in the morning, but store energy for the afternoon's activities, so one can have a little more for lunch. And at night, one is going to take a rest, so the amount of dinner should be relatively small.

------ 健康小提示 ------------------------------- **Health-preserving Tips**

晚餐应少吃,并选择好消化的食物,以稀粥为好,可以达到养胃、安神的作用。对于中老年人来说,可以吃些山药粥、莲子粥、红枣粥等。

One should eat less and choose digestible foods, such as porridge, which can also nourish the stomach and soothe the nerves. For middle-aged and elderly people, the porridge with Chinese yam, lotus or red dates is a good choice.

4 饥不暴食,渴不狂饮。

When being hungry, do not overeat; when being thirsty, do not over-drink.

所谓"饥不暴食,渴不狂饮"意指在很饿很渴的时候不要吃太多,喝太急。人在特别饥饿的状态下,脾胃虚弱,消化功能减弱。大量进食,会将食物滞留在肠胃内,造成肠胃饱胀。而在非常口渴的状态下,心脏以及肾脏的功能会减弱,大量饮水会使水分迅速进入血液,增加心脏和肾脏的负担,导致气血不平,易猝死。

The so-called "When being hungry, do not overeat; when being thirsty, do not overdrink" means not to eat too much or drink too quickly when one is very hungry and thirsty. When one is particularly hungry, his/her stomach and spleen are weak and the digestive functions are weakened. Eating a lot will make the food accumulate in the intestines and stomach and cause fullness. And in a very thirsty state, the function of the heart and kidneys will be weakened. Drinking a lot of water will cause water to quickly enter the bloodstream, increasing the burden on the heart and kidneys, leading to uneven blood and sudden death.

----- 健康小提示 ----------------------------- **Health-preserving Tips**

不要等到口渴的时候再喝水。真正口渴的时候,不要一气狂饮,要小口多饮。喝水量一次最好不要超过 300 毫升。尤其是在运动过后,不要剧烈饮水。

One should drink regularly before he/she feels very thirsty. When one is extremely thirsty, he/she shouldn't drink too much at a stretch but to drink more with sips. It is better not to drink more than 300ml at a time. Especially after exercise, one should not drink vigorously.

5 饭菜宜清淡,少盐少病患。
Meals should be light in that less salt reduces diseases.

这则谚语强调做饭时不宜在饭菜中放入太多的盐和调味品,人体摄入的盐分越少,生病的概率就越小。因此,口味偏重的人应逐步减少食用盐量。

This proverb emphasizes that it is not advisable to put too much salt and condiments in the food when cooking. The less salt the body consumes, the less chance of illness. Therefore, one with heavy taste should gradually reduce the amount of salt in diets.

----- 健康小提示 ----------------------------- **Health-preserving Tips**

炒菜时,少放盐,保留食物本身的味道。此外,可以多吃蔬菜、水果,因为蔬

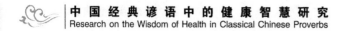

菜、水果能将盐中的钠排除到体外。

When cooking, one should put less salt to reserve the original taste of ingredients. In addition, one can eat more vegetables and fruit, which can remove the sodium in salt from the body.

6 生瓜梨枣，少吃为好。

It is good to eat less raw melons, pears and jujubes.

我国自古就有"生瓜梨枣，少吃为好"的说法，意思是即便是能生吃的瓜果，也要少吃一点。金元时代大医学家李杲说："内伤脾胃，百病由生。"在中医学上，瓜果类食物性凉，属寒，易伤脾胃。因此，中医常要求患者"忌凉"，以促进身体康复。

There has been a saying since ancient times that "It is good to eat less raw melons, pears and jujubes", which means that one should not eat more even though the melons and the fruits can be eaten raw. Li Gao, a great medical expert in the Jin and Yuan Dynasties, said："Internal damage in the stomach and the spleen causes diseases." In TCM, the melons and the fruits are cool in nature and pertain to cold food, and are prone to hurt the stomach and spleen. Therefore, TCM doctors generally require their patients that they are not supposed to eat cool food for the recovery.

------ 健康小提示 ------------------------------ **Health-preserving Tips**

冷饮易造成肠胃功能的紊乱，导致咽喉炎、支气管炎等呼吸道感染疾病。女性月经期喝冷饮容易引发宫寒，诱发痛经和月经不调等疾病。因此，应不喝或少喝冷饮。

Cold drinks can easily cause gastrointestinal disorders, leading to respiratory tract infections such as pharyngitis and bronchitis. Women during menstruation having cold drinks are prone to incur dysmenorrhea, irregular menstruation and other diseases. Drinking not or less is therefore rewarding for health.

7　美酒不过量，好菜不过食。

Good food is but food, and good wine is but wine.

　　宛光《河东谚》中说："美酒不过量，好菜不过食。"意思是说再好再香的酒，也不能贪杯；再好的菜，也不能贪吃。该句谚语强调饮酒吃菜都需适度，太过反而对身体不利。

　　Wan Guang said in *He Dong Yan* (*Proverbs in the East of the Yellow River*) that good food is but food, and good wine is but wine. It means that no matter how excellent the wine is, one cannot drink too much; no matter how delicious the food is, one cannot eat too much. This proverb emphasizes that drinking and eating must be moderate. Otherwise, it will do harm to the body.

------ **健康小提示** ------------------------------ **Health-preserving Tips**

　　饮酒要适度，尤其是酒量不行的人群更应少喝酒。饮酒时不宜过快，饮毕不要喝咖啡或者浓茶，因为咖啡会加重缺水状况，而茶叶会让身体处于一种兴奋状态。

　　Drinking should be moderate, especially one who cannot hold his/her drink. Don't drink too fast or have coffee or heavy tea after drinking, because coffee can aggravate the lack of water, and tea will make one excited.

8　吃盐莫过咸，吃糖只求甜。

Eating [less] salt for subtle salty taste; eating [less] sugar for subtle sweet taste.

　　盐和糖都是人们生活中的必需品，都有益于人，终生不食者不多，但过量食用盐和糖却有害于人，不可不知。中医上认为盐有消食、解毒、护胃之效，而养生的大法就是少调元气，因此吃东西的口味宜清淡。而吃糖过多会造成胃酸分泌过多，影响食欲，增加患糖尿病和肥胖病的风险。

　　Both salt and sugar are necessities in one's life, and they are good for everyone. There are few people who don't eat them. However, eating too much salt and sugar are harmful to people. In TCM, salt has the effects of promoting digestion, detoxifying, and nourishing the stomach. The fundamental method of health preservation is to stabilize the original *qi*, so the food should be light. Eating too much sugar may cause excessive gastric acid secretion, affect appetite, and increase the risk of obesity and diabetes.

------ 健康小提示 ------------------------------------ **Health-preserving Tips**

食盐过多会导致人反应变慢,口渴频繁,局部水肿。因此,肾脏病人、肝硬化腹水病人、心力衰竭病人以及高血压病人不能吃太多盐。

Too much salt causes slower reactions, frequent thirst and local edema. Therefore, patients suffering from kidney disease, cirrhosis and ascites, heart failure and hypertension should not eat too much salt.

9 红薯贱物,不宜多吃。
Sweet potatoes are cheap, but one should not eat more.

民间有谚语:红薯贱物,不宜多吃。意思是红薯价格便宜,但不能因便宜就过多食用。中医认为"甘薯补虚,健脾开胃,强肾阴"。红薯本身富含蛋白质、纤维素、维生素及多种矿物质,对人体健康有益。但生吃或多吃反而不利于健康,其高含糖量易导致胃酸过多、恶心反胃。

Sweet potatoes are cheap, but one should not eat more. It means that although sweet potatoes are cheap, one should not eat too much because of low price. TCM holds that sweet potatoes tonify deficiency, invigorate the spleen and increase the appetite, and strengthen the kidney *yin*. Sweet potatoes are rich in protein, fibre, vitamins and various minerals, which are beneficial to human health. However, eating raw or eating more is not good for health because its high sugar content can easily cause hyperacidity and nausea.

------ 健康小提示 ------------------------------------ **Health-preserving Tips**

红薯不宜空腹食用,否则会导致胃酸过多;红薯不宜和柿子同食,其糖分易和柿子中的果胶发生反应,增加胃溃疡的发病率。

Do not eat sweet potatoes on an empty stomach, because they are prone to cause excessive stomach acid. Do not eat sweet potatoes with persimmon because their sugar can easily react with the pectin in persimmon to increase the incidence of gastric ulcer.

10　贪吃贪睡,添病减岁。

Being greedy for eating and sleeping makes one sick and short-lived.

吃和睡是人的自然本能。谚语"贪吃贪睡, 添病减岁"告诫人们吃得多、睡得多,不利于健康长寿,强调适量饮食及睡眠的重要性。因为长期长时间的睡眠会导致新陈代谢缓慢,肠胃功能紊乱,胃黏膜受到损害以及体内能量消耗不足;贪吃容易导致食道和胃部急性扩张,引发急性肠胃炎等疾病。

Eating and sleeping are human instincts. The proverb "Being greedy for eating and sleeping makes one sick and short-lived" warns people that over-eating and over-sleeping are not conducive to health and longevity. It emphasizes the importance of proper diet and sleep. Because long-term sleep will lead to slow metabolism, gastrointestinal dysfunction, gastric mucosa damage and insufficient energy consumption in the body; gluttony leads to acute dilatation of the stomach and esophagus, causing acute gastroenteritis and other diseases.

------ 健康小提示 ----------------------------- **Health-preserving Tips**

人们在做菜时,尽量少油少盐少糖少辣,这样不会特别刺激食欲。睡前要关门关窗以防感染风寒。每天适当睡午觉,既温补阳气,又可以健脾胃。

One should use less oil, salt, sugar and chili, so that his/her appetite is not stimulated. Before going to bed, one should close doors and windows to prevent infection of wind and cold. It is better to take a proper nap every day, which can not only warm and tonify *yang qi*, but also nourish the stomach and spleen.

11 饮食有节,起居有常,劳逸有度。

Moderate in eating and drinking, regular in daily life, and balanced in working and resting are good for health preservation.

《黄帝内经》谈健康时说道:"饮食有节,起居有常,劳逸有度。"意思是食饮要有节制,起居要有规律,不过度操劳。该句谚语强调了遵循自然界规律的重要性,如此便能健康长寿。

As the saying in *Huang Di Nei Jing* (*Huangdi's Canon of Medicine*) goes, "Moderate in eating and drinking, regular in daily life and balanced in working and resting are good for health preservation." The proverb means that one must be restrained in eating and drinking, the individual life should be regular, and overwork should be avoided. This proverb emphasizes the importance of following the natural laws so as to live a long and healthy life.

------ 健康小提示 ----------------------------- **Health-preserving Tips**

饮食上,食物搭配要合理多样,切忌暴饮暴食或偏食;起居上,遵循"春夏养阳,秋冬养阴"的原则";工作上,无论多忙也要注意适当休息。

One should eat variously and overeating should be avoided. In sleep, one should obey the principle of "nourishing *yang* in spring and summer while nourishing *yin* in autumn and winter". One should also take a good rest even he/she is very busy.

12 橘子温热能养人,多吃吃错惹祸根。

The tangerine is warm-hot in nature and can nourish human body, but eating it too much is harmful.

这则谚语强调吃橘子要适度。中医认为橙子性温,属热,多吃易患内热,尤其是阴虚阳亢的人最好少吃橘子。因此,风寒咳嗽、痰饮咳嗽者不宜食用橘子。

This proverb emphasizes that one should eat tangerines in moderation. TCM holds that tangerines are warm in nature and pertain to heat food. If eating more, people are prone to internal heat, especially those with *yin* deficiency and *yang* hyperactivity. One suffering from cold cough and phlegm cough should eat less.

吃橘子前后 1 小时不要喝牛奶,这是由于牛奶中的蛋白质碰到果酸会凝结,影响消化吸收。

Do not drink milk for one hour before or after eating tangerines. This is because the protein in milk will coagulate when it encounters fruit acids, which will affect digestion and absorption.

13　勿使悲欢极,当令饮食均。

Grief and joy should not be extreme, while diet should be balanced.

唐代著名大医药学家孙思邈在《养生要集》中说:"勿使悲欢极,当令饮食均。"该句说明要保持健康的生活方式,生活起居一定要有规律,饮食要节制,膳食要平衡。

Sun Simiao said in the book *Yang Sheng Yao Ji* (*A Collection of Health Preservation*), "Grief and joy should not be extreme, while diet should be balanced." This sentence indicates that to maintain a healthy lifestyle, daily life must be regular, diet must be moderate and balanced.

夜间不要大吃大喝和酒醉,以免引起停食、消化不良或伤胃、伤肝等不良后果。

Do not overeat and overdrink at night and get drunk to avoid adverse consequences such as dyspepsia, indigestion or stomach and liver injury.

14　食无求饱,五脏即安。

Do not seek for fullness when one has food, and the five *zang* viscera will be peaceful.

饮食是人体赖以生存、保持健康的必要条件,又是导致疾病发生的重要原因之一。《论语》中说:"食无求饱,居无求安。"就是说,饮食节制,人体脏腑就会处于安宁的状态中。

Diet is a necessary condition for the human body to survive and maintain health, and it is also one of the important causes of disease. A saying in *Lun Yu* (*The Analects*) goes that "Do not seek for fullness when one has food, and the five *zang* viscera will be peaceful." That is to say, if one practices temperance in eating and drinking, the five *zang* viscera and six *fu* viscera will be peaceful.

----- 健康小提示 ------------------------------- **Health-preserving Tips**

平日里饮食吃七八分饱即可。节食的人应注意饮食不能太过节制,否则营养摄入量不足,会导致气血乏源、五脏受损。

In general, seventy to eighty percent of fullness is enough. One who is dieting must note that controlling diet should not be extreme, otherwise the absorbed nutrition will be insufficient, which causes lack of source of *qi* and blood, and damages the five *zang* viscera.

15　瓜果虽美,不可多尝。

Although melons and fruits are delicious, do not eat too much.

瓜果是人们饭桌之余的必备品。一到暑季,天气炎热,人们进食瓜果的次数就会增加,尤其是冷藏过的水果都是人们爱吃的东西。古谚"瓜果虽美,不可多尝"即是说瓜果的味道虽然好,但大多属凉,性寒,不宜多吃。吃多了会增加肠胃的负担,引起消化问题。

Melons and fruits are a must-have for people besides the meals. In the summer, as the weather is hot, one will eat more melons and fruits, especially fruits that have been refrigerated are what one likes very much. The old saying "Although melons and fruits are delicious, do not eat too much" refers that melons and fruits are sweet, but they are cool in nature, so it is not suitable for one to have more. Eating too much increases the burden on the stomach and causes digestive problems.

----- 健康小提示 ------------------------------ **Health-preserving Tips**

吃水果宜在饭前半小时,这样可以降低糖类摄入的含量。但是柿子、香蕉、橘子、山楂、甘蔗、鲜荔枝等水果,不宜空腹时吃,否则不利于身体健康。

It is advisable to eat fruits half an hour before meals, which can lower the content of sugar intake. But some kinds of fruits, such as persimmons, bananas, tangerines, hawthorns, sugar cane and fresh litchi, should not be eaten on an empty stomach, otherwise it is not good for health.

16　茶喝多了养性,酒喝多了伤身。

Drinking too much tea cultivates one's temperament, while drinking too much alcohol hurts one's body.

民间有谚语"茶喝多了养性,酒喝多了伤身"。意思是说茶味清爽,喝多了能静心养性;酒性浓烈,喝多了有害身体。本谚语强调经常喝茶有益,过量喝酒有害。中医认为上午阳气开始生发,喝绿茶,有升清作用,能使一天神清气爽。

A folk proverb says that drinking too much tea cultivates one's temperament, while drinking too much alcohol hurts one's body. It means that the tea is refreshing, and if one drinks it often, the heart can calm down and the body will get nourishment; the alcohol is strong, and if one drinks too much, it is harmful to the body. It emphasizes that drinking tea regularly is beneficial, but excessive alcohol is harmful. And in TCM, in the morning, *yang qi* begins to grow, and drinking green tea has the effect of ascending the clear and descending the turbid.

----- 健康小提示 ------------------------------ **Health-preserving Tips**

中医认为人的体质有燥热、虚寒之别。燥热体质的人,应喝凉性茶,如绿茶;虚寒体质者,应喝温性茶,如红茶、普洱茶。

TCM believes that human physique can be divided into dryness-heat and deficiency-cold. People with hot constitution should drink tea with cool nature, like green tea. People with deficiency and cold constitution should drink tea with warm nature, such as black tea and Pu'er tea.

17 会吃千顿香,乱吃一顿伤。

Eating with regular diet is beneficial; eating without limitation causes diseases.

古谚"会吃千顿香,乱吃一顿伤",不是说人会吃,顿顿都吃得香,而是指饮食有节制,顿顿才会吃得香;暴饮暴食,一次就会大伤脾胃,危害身体健康。

The old saying "Eating with regular diet is beneficial; eating without limitation causes diseases" does not mean that one enjoys every meal if he/she knows how to have a meal better, but means that one enjoys every meal if he/she has a meal with limitation. Furthermore, if one is crapulent, only one meal will damage the stomach and spleen greatly, and do harm to the body.

------ 健康小提示 ---------------------------- **Health-preserving Tips**

中医认为,早餐应该吃热食,以保护胃气。因为早上人体内的神经及血管都还处于收缩状态,此时如果吃冰冷的食品,可能使消化系统发生痉挛。

TCM holds that one should eat warm food in the morning, so as to protect the stomach *qi*. Because the nerves and blood vessels in the human body are still in a state of contraction in the morning, if one eats cold food at this time, it may cause the spasm of digestive system.

18 少饮健体,多饮伤身。

Drinking less (alcohol) builds up one's body while drinking more hurts one's body.

中国的饮食文化与酒息息相关。酒喝对了能促进血液循环,有益身体健康,消除疲劳,抵抗寒冷。但凡事皆有两面,过量饮酒会对大脑神经造成损害,危害肝脏,进而威胁健康。所谓"少饮健体,多饮伤身"告诉我们,适量饮酒有益健康,饮酒过多则有损健康。

Chinese food culture is closely related to wine. Drinking correctly can promote blood circulation, benefit one's health, relieve the fatigue and resist the cold. But everything has two sides. Excessive drinking does harm to the nerves and brain, damages the liver, and threatens one's health. The so-called "Drinking less alcohol builds up one's body while drinking more hurts one's body" tells us that drinking in moderation is good for one's health, while drinking too much is harmful to our health.

----- **健康小提示** -------------------------------- **Health-preserving Tips**

不要空腹喝酒,喝酒前不可大量饮水;喝酒时忌饮用冰水、柠檬水等刺激性的饮料。

Do not drink on an empty stomach, and do not drink a lot of water before drinking. When drinking, do not drink stimulating beverages such as ice water and lemonade.

第二节　药食同源
Section Two　Homology of Medicine and Food

1　大蒜是个宝,常吃身体好。
Garlic is a treasure and regular eating is good to human body.

大蒜是一种调味品,也是一种中药。从中医学角度来讲,大蒜性温、味辛,可以温中止痛、行气、解毒杀虫。吃了大蒜可以有效地缓解腹泻、痢疾,还可以杀灭一些寄生虫、改善外阴瘙痒等症状,是一种不错的保健食品。因而民间常说"大蒜是个宝,常吃身体好"。

Garlic is not only a kind of food seasoning, but also a kind of Chinese medicinal. From the perspective of TCM, garlic is warm in nature and pungent in taste, which can warm the middle and relieve pain, promote *qi*, remove toxin and kill parasites. Eating garlic can effectively relieve diarrhea and dysentery, and can also kill parasites and cure pruritus vulvae. So it is a good health food. Therefore, people often say that "Garlic is a treasure and regular eating is good to human body."

------ **健康小提示** ----------------------------- **Health-preserving Tips**

夏季湿气重，多吃蒜可以除湿邪，但秋冬季节干燥，容易上火，最好少吃。对于体质虚弱和胃肠衰弱的人，可以适当吃些熟蒜，减少大蒜素对肠胃的刺激。

In summer, the humidity is heavy, and eating more garlic can remove dampness pathogen. But in autumn and winter, the weather is dry and one is easy to get inner heat, so it is better to eat less garlic. For people with weak physique and gastrointestinal weakness, they can eat some cooked garlic, which can effectively reduce the irritation of garlic to the stomach.

2 要想人长寿，多吃豆腐少吃肉。

If one wants to live longer, eat more tofu and less meat.

豆腐是汉代刘安发明的美味食品，广受中国人的喜爱。谚语"要想人长寿，多吃豆腐少吃肉"告诉我们豆腐营养价值高，生活当中应适当多次食用。相对来说，适当少吃一些肉，有利于健康长寿。中医学上，豆腐味甘性凉，具有益气、生津润燥、清热解毒的功效。但是需注意，这里的"多吃"强调的是少食多次。

Tofu is a delicious food made by Liu An in the Han Dynasty and is widely popular in China. The proverb "If one wants to live longer, eat more tofu and less meat" tells us that tofu has high nutritional value, so it is better to eat tofu more often and eat less meat. This is beneficial to health and longevity. In TCM, tofu is sweet and is cool in nature, and has the effects of replenishing *qi*, promoting body fluid and moistening dryness, clearing heat and relieving toxin. But it should be noted that "eat more" here does not mean eating much at a time but eating it several more times.

------ **健康小提示** ----------------------------- **Health-preserving Tips**

豆腐虽然营养丰富，但缺乏膳食纤维，单独吃可能会带来便秘的麻烦。而青菜和木耳中都含有丰富的膳食纤维，正好能弥补豆腐的这一缺点。另外，木耳和青菜还含有许多能提高免疫力、预防疾病的抗氧化成分，搭配豆腐食用，抗病作用更好。

Although tofu is rich in nutrients, it lacks in dietary fiber. Eating alone may cause constipation. And green vegetables and wood ear are rich in dietary fiber, which can make up for the shortcoming of tofu. In addition, wood ear and green vegetables also contain many antioxidants that can improve immunity and prevent diseases. The effect of disease resistance is better when one eats them with tofu.

3　白菜吃半年,医生享清闲。
Eating Chinese cabbage for half a year keeps the doctor away.

在我国流传着"白菜吃半年,医生享清闲"的谚语,强调了白菜的营养价值。

生活中,白菜作为食材广为人知,但白菜还具有一定的药用价值。中医上讲,大白菜味甘、性平,可通利肠胃,去除胸中烦闷。

There is a proverb in our country that goes, "Eating Chinese cabbage for half a year keeps the doctor away." The proverb emphasizes the nutritional value of Chinese cabbage. In people's daily life, Chinese cabbage is widely known as an ingredient, but it also has certain medicinal value. In TCM, Chinese cabbage is sweet in taste and neutral in nature, which can promote urination and remove the irritation.

----- 健康小提示 ---------------------------------- **Health-preserving Tips**

在日常生活中要多吃白菜,常吃白菜,有利于预防和治疗疾病。

It is better to eat more Chinese cabbage in daily life. Eating it frequently is beneficial to the prevention and treatment of diseases.

4　朝食三片姜,犹如人参汤。
Eating some slices of ginger in the morning is like drinking ginseng soup.

老话说:"朝食三片姜,胜过人参汤。"意思是说,在早上吃三片姜,保健的作用比人参汤还好。姜是一种食物调味品,具有神奇的保健功效。每天早晨喝一

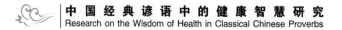

些姜汤,发汗解表,排出毒素,对提高人体抗病力有帮助。

As the old saying goes, "Eating some slices of ginger in the morning is like drinking ginseng soup." It means that eating three slices of ginger in the morning is better than ginseng soup in health preservation. Ginger is a kind of food seasoning with magical health effects. Drinking some ginger soup every morning to induce sweating to release the exterior and dispel toxins is beneficial to improve the body's disease resistance.

----- **健康小提示** ----------------------------- **Health-preserving Tips**

姜是温性食物,容易上火,所以不宜食用过多,否则会伤阴助阳。生姜腐烂时一定不能食用,因为烂姜中有黄樟素能致肝癌或食道癌。

Ginger is warm in nature and is prone to cause heat, so one should not eat too much. Otherwise, it will damage *yin* and strengthen *yang*. One should not eat rotten ginger, because there is safrol in it that leads to liver cancer or esophageal cancer.

5　天天吃醋,年年无灾。

Having vinegar every day, keeping healthy every year.

"天天吃醋,年年无灾",这条民谚说出了醋有利于人体健康。醋是一种食药两用的药材:作为食材是一种很好的调味品;作为药材可以用来治病救人。醋不仅能刺激人的胃口,增强食欲,还具有抗菌解毒、降低血压的功效。

The proverb "Having vinegar every day, keeping healthy every year" shows that vinegar is good for human health. Vinegar is a kind of medicinal material that belongs to food and medicine. As food, it is a good condiment; as an ingredient, it can be used to cure some diseases. It can not only stimulate one's appetite, but also have the effects of killing germ, removing toxin and lowering blood pressure.

----- **健康小提示** ----------------------------- **Health-preserving Tips**

在日常生活中可以多食醋,但并不是适用于所有人。比如胃酸过多、骨质疏松者不宜多食醋。

One can eat vinegar several more times in daily life, but it is not suitable for everyone. For example, people with hyperacidity and osteoporosis should not eat more vinegar.

6　多吃芹菜不用问，降低血压很管用。
Eating celery often is helpful for lowering blood pressure.

"多吃芹菜不用问，降低血压很管用"确实有凭有据，而在中医看来，芹菜具有清热除烦、平肝调经、利水解毒、凉血消肿、止血之功效。民间用新鲜芹菜捣汁饮服，或用芹菜根煎水饮，每次一茶杯，每日二次，对降血压有效果。据报道，现在已有研究部门将旱芹制成酊剂，或从芹菜中提炼出芹菜碱，用来治疗高血压，效果很好。

It is evident that eating celery often is helpful for lowering blood pressure. In TCM, celery has the effects of clearing heat and eliminating irritability, pacifying liver and regulating menstruation, inducing diuresis and removing toxin, cooling blood to alleviate edema and stop bleeding. To lower blood pressure, people often drink fresh celery juice, or drink soup made from the roots of celery. Have one cup of the juice each time, twice a day, the effect is remarkable. According to reports, medical research departments have turned dried celery to tinctures, or extracted celery alkali from it, which is used to treat high blood pressure with very good results.

----- 健康小提示 ---------------------------------- **Health-preserving Tips**

脾胃虚寒的人群不宜吃芹菜，低血压人群不宜吃芹菜，吃芹菜时不要放醋，芹菜不能与蛤蜊一起吃。

People with poor stomach and spleen should not eat celery. People with low blood pressure should not eat celery. Do not add vinegar in celery, and do not eat it with clams.

7 常吃葱，人轻松。

Eating green onion often makes one feel relaxed.

葱在我们的日常生活当中是一种普遍的调味品或蔬菜。其实葱除了用作烹饪食材外，对人体健康也有诸多好处。谚语"常吃葱，人轻松"强调了多吃葱的好处。中医学上讲，葱能够发汗解表，具有健胃功效，可提高食欲，增强体质。

Green onion is a common condiment or vegetable in one's daily life. In fact, green onions are not only used as cooking ingredients, but also have many benefits to human health. The proverb "Eating green onion often makes one feel relaxed" emphasizes the benefits of eating onions. In TCM, green onion induces sweating to release the exterior and strengthen the stomach, which can increase appetite and enhance the physique.

------ 健康小提示 ------------------------------ **Health-preserving Tips**

吃葱虽好，但也不易过量，否则会引起头昏、视物不清。感冒的病人可以多吃葱，帮助出汗。另外，葱不能和蜂蜜同时食用。

Although eating green onions is good, one should not eat too much, otherwise it will cause dizziness and blurred vision. Patients with common cold can eat more green onions to induce sweat. In addition, green onions cannot be eaten with honey at the same time.

8 常吃一点醋，不用去药铺。

Eating a little vinegar often will keep one away from drug stores.

醋多为粮食发酵而成，味酸，是日常饮食中经常用到的调味品。其实醋中含有种类多样的氨基酸等营养物质，不仅能够补充身体所需营养，而且可以软化血管、疏通气血、健脾开胃等。

Vinegar is mostly fermented from grains and tastes sour. It is a seasoning often used in diet. Actually, vinegar contains a variety of nutrients such as amino acids, which can not only supplement the nutrients needed by the body, but also soften blood vessels, free the *qi* and blood and invigorate the spleen and stomach.

------ **健康小提示** ---------------------------- **Health-preserving Tips**

醋偏酸,如果食用过多,人的体质容易变成酸性体质,引起胃炎。

Vinegar is meta-acid. Having too much vinegar will lead to acid physique and gastritis.

9　多吃豆,能长寿。

Eating more beans promotes one to live longer.

谚语"多吃豆,能长寿"强调了豆类食品对人体健康的促进作用。豆类食物品种繁多,常见的有黄豆、绿豆、豌豆等。在所有的豆类植物中,黄豆的蛋白质含量是最高的,而且黄豆中含有多种人体需要的氨基酸,所以多吃黄豆或者黄豆制成的食品对我们健康是有好处的。

The proverb "Eating more beans promotes one to live longer" emphasizes the contribution of bean products to human health. There are many kinds of bean products. Some common ones are soybeans, mung beans and peas. Among these beans, soybean contains the highest protein. It has a variety of amino acids that human body needs, so eating more soybeans or foods made from soybeans is good for people's health.

------ **健康小提示** ---------------------------- **Health-preserving Tips**

豆制品虽然好处大,可是也不可一次食用过多,否则对肠胃有伤害!

Although soy products have great benefits, one cannot eat too much at one time. Overeating is harmful to intestines and stomach.

10　常饮菊花茶,老来不眼花。

Drinking chrysanthemum tea often can prevent one from getting presbyopia in the old age.

菊花茶,是一种以菊花为原料制成的花草茶。据古籍记载,菊花味甘苦,性耐寒,有散风清热、清肝明目和解毒消炎等作用。因此,常常喝菊花茶不易导致花眼。

Chrysanthemum tea is a kind of herbal tea made from chrysanthemum. According to ancient records, chrysanthemum tastes sweet and bitter, is cold-tolerant in nature, has the effects of dispersing wind and clearing heat, clearing liver and improving vision, and can remove toxin to eliminate inflammation. Therefore, drinking chrysanthemum tea more often can reduce the risk of suffering from presbyopia.

------ 健康小提示 ----------------------------------- **Health-preserving Tips**

喝茶要随泡随饮。菊花茶中富含黄酮类物质,但黄酮类物质十分不稳定,很容易被氧化,使茶水失去本来的黄色色泽,变成绿色,其保健作用也会有所下降。

Drink tea immediately after having made it. Chrysanthemum tea is rich in flavonoids. But it is very unstable and is easily oxidized, causing the tea to lose its original color and turn green. At this time, the health-preserving effect will also be reduced.

11 日日吃三枣,一辈子不见老。
Eat three dates every day, and one never knows how old he/she is.

本句谚语强调了大枣的养生保健功效。"日日吃三枣"不是说每天吃三颗枣,这里的"三"只是强调每天吃一些枣。"一辈子不见老"是说大枣具有滋阴补阳的功效,经常食用对皮肤好。中医学上也认为大枣是补中益气、养血安神的佳品,其枣仁和根均为重要药品。

This proverb emphasizes the health-preserving effect of dates. "Eat three dates every day" does mean eating some dates every day. "One never knows how old he/she is" refers that the date has the effect of nourishing *yin* and *yang*, so regular eating is good for the skin. In TCM, date is also considered to be a good product for tonifying middle and replenishing *qi*, nourishing blood and inducing tranquilization. Both its seeds and roots are important medicines.

------ 健康小提示 ----------------------------------- **Health-preserving Tips**

人在生活当中可以喝一些大枣莲子粥:大枣 10 枚,山药 30 克,莲子 15 克,

大米 100 克。早晚食用,效果更佳。

People can drink porridge with dates and lotus seed in daily life: made with 10 dates, 30 grams of yam, 15 grams of lotus seeds, and 100 grams of rice. Have the porridge in the morning and evening is much better.

12 核桃山中宝,补肾又健脑。

Walnuts, the treasure on the mountain, invigorate human brain and tonify human spleen.

古往今来民间一直有"以形补形"的说法。因为核桃看起来状似人脑,所以人们多认为吃核桃可以补脑。从中医学角度来讲,核桃味甘、性温,可入肾、肺、大肠经,故而有补肾固精、润肺定喘、润肠通便、健胃补血的功效,所以常吃核桃可以有效缓解阳痿遗精、小便频数、大便燥结等不适。

Throughout the ages, there has been a saying among the people that "one benefits from what he/she eats". Because walnuts look like human brains, one thinks that eating walnuts can replenish the brain. From the perspective of TCM, walnut tastes sweet and is warm in nature. It enters kidney channel, lung channel and large intestine channel, so it has the effects of tonifying kidney and securing essence, moistening lung to arrest panting, moistening intestines to relieve constipation, and invigorating stomach and tonifying blood. Eating walnuts often can effectively alleviate diseases, such as impotence, frequent urination and dry stool.

------ 健康小提示 ------------------------------- **Health-preserving Tips**

核桃是很好的补品。不过要注意,食用过多容易生内热,所以每天早或晚各吃 1 或 2 个最为适宜。

Walnut is a good tonic. However, it should be noted that eating too much is easy to cause internal heat, so it is most appropriate to eat one or two in the morning or evening.

13 鼻子不通,吃点大葱。

[If you] have a stuffy nose, eat some green Chinese onion.

《本草纲目》中说,葱性味辛平、甘温,能治寒热和肝中邪气。在我国民间,感冒鼻塞时,用葱段加姜片煮一碗汤,趁热喝下去,再盖上被子出点汗,感冒的症状就会减轻或痊愈。医学证明,葱不仅能刺激汗腺,有发汗解表的作用,还具有较强的杀菌作用。

The book, *Ben Cao Gang Mu* (*Compendium of Materia Medica*), points out that green onion is neutral in nature, and is acrid in taste. It can cure fever and chills and liver pathogen. In our country, when one catches a cold and has a stuffy nose, he/she often takes in a bowl of soup cooked with a few pieces of green onions and ginger slices, and covers the body with a quilt to induce a little sweat. Then, the symptoms of the cold will be relieved or healed. It is medically proven that green onions can stimulate sweat glands, have the effect of induce sweating to release superficies, and also have a strong germ-killing effect.

------ 健康小提示 ----------------------------------- **Health-preserving Tips**

患有肠胃疾病的人不建议过多食用大葱,避免对肠胃产生刺激。

Patients with gastrointestinal diseases are not recommended to eat too much green Chinese onions to avoid irritation to the stomach.

14 若要不失眠,煮粥加白莲。

If one wants to avoid insomnia, he/she can[eat] porridge with some white lotus.

民间常说:"若要不失眠,煮粥加白莲。"这里的白莲就是指莲子,它归脾、肾、心经络,有养心安神的功效,对虚烦惊悸、失眠等症特别有效。当代科学研究证实,莲籽除带有多种营养元素外,还带有荷叶碱,对神经衰弱病症有非常好的改进功效。

People often say, "If one wants to avoid insomnia, he/she can[eat] porridge with some white lotus." The white lotus refers to lotus seed, which enters to the spleen channel, kidney channel and heart meridians, and has the effect of nourishing heart and inducing tranquilization. It is especially effective for treating symptoms such as vacuity vexation, fright palpitations, and insomnia. Contemporary scientific research has confirmed that in addition to a variety of nutrients, lotus seed also contains nuciferine, which is very good to improve neurasthenia.

------ 健康小提示 --------------------------------- **Health-preserving Tips**

莲子粥制法：莲子与稻米、小米或糯米一同放入锅中，温火炖烂。煮好的莲子粥能够放进冷藏室，每天晚饭时加温服用。

Recipe of lotus seed porridge：Put some lotus seeds and rice, millet or glutinous rice into a pot and then simmer them by gentle heat. The cooked lotus seed porridge can be put in the refrigerator and warmed up at dinner every day.

15　常把核桃吃，润肤黑发须。

Eating walnuts often can moisten one's skin and make one's hair black.

民间认为吃核桃不仅补脑，还能滋养头发。核桃中 86% 的脂肪是不饱和脂肪酸，富含铜、镁、钾以及多种维生素。中医学同样认为，核桃具有润肌肤、乌黑须发的功效。

People believe that eating walnuts not only nourishes the brain, but also nourishes the hair. 86% of fat in walnuts is unsaturated fatty acids, which are rich in copper, magnesium, potassium and other vitamins. TCM also holds that walnuts have the effects of moisturizing the skin and making hair black.

------ 健康小提示 --------------------------------- **Health-preserving Tips**

秋冬季是吃核桃的最佳时季。连续几个月吃核桃，可以乌黑头发。每天吃 2 个就足够了。

It is best to eat walnuts in autumn and winter. Eating walnuts for several months can make one's hair black. It is enough to eat two every day.

16 明目找菊花，补血玫瑰茶。

Drinking chrysanthemum tea can improve vision, drinking rose tea can tonify blood.

本谚语强调了菊花和玫瑰的药用疗法。菊花是一味中药，古人把菊花称为"延寿客"。菊花味甘苦，性耐寒，有散风清热、清肝明目和解毒消炎等作用。玫瑰花含有丰富的维生素，能调气血、促进血液循环。

This proverb emphasizes the medicinal treatments of chrysanthemums and roses. Chrysanthemum is a traditional Chinese medicine. The ancients called chrysanthemum "the guest of longevity". Chrysanthemum tastes sweet and bitter, is cold-tolerant in nature, and has the effects of dispersing wind and clearing heat, clearing liver and improving vision, and can remove toxin to eliminate inflammation. Roses are rich in vitamins, which can regulate *qi* and blood and promote blood circulation.

----- 健康小提示 ----------------------------- **Health-preserving Tips**

玫瑰花茶有收敛的作用，便秘患者不宜饮用。同时，玫瑰花茶具有比较强的活血散瘀的功效，因此经期血量多的女性在月经期间要少喝或者不喝。

Rose tea has the effect of astringency, so patients with constipation should not drink it. At the same time, rose tea has a relatively strong effect of activating blood to dissipate stasis, so women with high blood volume during menstruation should drink less or not.

17 口渴心烦躁，粥加猕猴桃。

If one feels thirsty and irritable, [eat] porridge with kiwi fruit.

民间常说"口渴心烦躁，粥加猕猴桃"，意思是说若我们感到口渴心烦，可以食用猕猴桃粥，即在粥中加入猕猴桃同时烹饪。中医学认为，猕猴桃性寒，味甘，具有调中理气、清热解暑、生津止渴、健胃消食的功效。因此，心易躁动的人可以在食用的粥中加入适当的猕猴桃。

People often say that if one feels thirsty and irritable, 〔eat〕 porridge with kiwi fruit, which means that if feeling thirsty and upset, people can have kiwi porridge. In TCM, kiwi fruit is cold in nature, sweet in taste, and has the effects of regulating the middle and *qi*, clearing the heat and releasing the summerheat, engendering fluid to quench thirst, and invigorating stomach to promote digestion. Therefore, one who is easily restless can add some kiwi fruit to his/her porridge.

----- **健康小提示** ------------------------------ **Health-preserving Tips**

猕猴桃性寒,女性在经期不宜食用猕猴桃;食用猕猴桃不宜过量,1~2个就足够了;不要空腹食用。

Kiwi fruit is cold in nature, so women should not eat it during menstruation. Do not eat it too much at one time. One or two kiwi fruit are enough. Do not eat on an empty stomach.

18　常用五香粉,少登医院门。
Often use five spice powder, and skip doctor visits.

五香粉,是指将超过5种的香料研磨成粉,再混合在一起的调味料,常涂抹在煎、炸前的鸡、鸭肉类上,也可与细盐混合做蘸料食用。五香粉汇集了各种原料的优点,气味芳香,具辛温之性,有健脾温中、消炎利尿等功效,对提高机体抵抗力有一定帮助。

Five spice powder refers to a seasoning made by grinding over five kinds of spices into powder and then mixing them together. It is often used to apply to chicken and duck meat before frying, or it can be mixed with fine salt to make a dipping sauce. Five spice powder combines the advantages of various raw materials, has a fragrant smell, is pungent and warm in nature. It has the effects of invigorating spleen and warming the middle, and eliminating inflammation to promote urination, and is helpful to improve the body's immunity.

----- **健康小提示** ------------------------------ **Health-preserving Tips**

五香粉使用时应以少为宜,因为其中所含的桂皮、丁香、茴香、生姜以及胡椒

等料虽然属于天然调味品,但若用量过多,同样具有一定的副作用乃至毒性和诱变性。

The dosage of five spice powder should be less because the contained ingredients, such as cinnamon, *dingxiang* (clove), *huixiang* (fennel), *shengjiang* (fresh ginger) and *hujiao* (pepper fruit), are natural spices. Over-dosage has side effects and even has toxic effects.

19 空心莲菜凉,有病无病只管尝。

The hollow lotus root is cold in nature. It is good to eat for the sick or the healthy.

这则谚语是我国劳动人民长期生活实践的经验总结,基本符合中医学的食疗原理。莲,质白而中空,古时常为人们食用,故视作蔬菜的一种。莲菜亦食亦药。中医学认为,莲菜性凉,有消瘀凉血、清烦热的功效。

This proverb is the summary of experience of our working people's long-term life practice, which basically conforms to the dietary principles of Chinese medicine. The lotus is white and hollow. People had it in the past, so it is also regarded as a kind of vegetable. Lotus can be used as food and medicine. In TCM, lotus is cool in nature, and has the effects of dissipating stasis, cooling blood, and clearing vexing heat.

------ 健康小提示 ------------------------------ **Health-preserving Tips**

作为食物和药物,莲菜在我们日常生活中发挥着不可或缺的作用,但体质寒凉者不宜多食。

As food and medicine, lotus plays an indispensable role in our daily lives. It is not suitable for people with cold constitution to eat it.

20 鸡蛋生喝,润喉清热。

Eating raw eggs can soothe the throat and clear the heat.

鸡蛋不仅是一种常见食材,也是一味良药,其药用价值较高。在中医处方中,鸡蛋的不同部位被称为鸡子白(蛋清)、鸡子黄(蛋黄)、蛋壳(蛋皮)和蛋膜衣。鸡蛋滋阴润燥、镇心益气,有多种功效,性平、微寒、无毒、味甘。生喝鸡蛋可起到润喉清热的效果。

Egg is not only a common ingredient, but also a good medicine with high medicinal value. In traditional Chinese medicine prescriptions, different parts of eggs are called *ji zi bai* (egg white), *ji zi huang* (egg yolk), egg shell (egg skin) and egg film. Egg nourishes *yin*, moistens dryness, calms heart and nourishes *qi*, and is neutral and mildly cold in nature. Moreover, it is non-toxic and tastes sweet. Eating raw eggs can soothe the throat and clear the heat.

----- 健康小提示 ----------------------------- **Health-preserving Tips**

可以根据个人的症状选择鸡蛋的不同部位服用。

One can choose different parts of the egg to take according to his/her symptoms.

21 饥时荔枝,饱食黄皮。

Being hungry to eat litchi and being full to eat wampee.

在我国广东地区有"饥时荔枝,饱食黄皮"一说,意思是饥饿时可吃荔枝充饥,饱胀时可吃黄皮来消食。中医学认为荔枝味甘,性温,入心、脾、肝经,具有补脾益肝、理气补血、温中止痛的功效;而黄皮果具有促进消化、顺气镇咳、消暑生津的功效。

In Guangdong, China, there is a proverb that goes, "Being hungry to eat litchi and being full to eat wampee." In TCM, litchi is sweet in taste and warm in nature, enters the heart channel, spleen channel and liver channel, and has the effects of tonifying the spleen and liver, regulating *qi* and tonifying blood, warming the middle and relieving pain. Wampee has the effects of promoting digestion, smoothing *qi*, settling cough, and clearing summerheat and engendering fluid.

----- 健康小提示 ----------------------------- **Health-preserving Tips**

荔枝性温,吃多易上火,故不适合阴虚和湿热体质人群食用。黄皮果性凉,

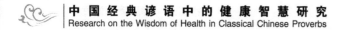
所以不适合脾胃虚寒的人或患有胃炎的人食用。

Litchi is warm in nature. Eating it too much will be prone to produce internal heat, so it is not suitable for one with *yin* deficiency and damp-heat constitution. Wampee is cold in nature. People with poor spleen and stomach or people suffering from gastritis should not to eat it.

22 血虚夜不眠，米粥煨桂圆。

Having rice porridge with dried longan (*Dimocarpus longan Lour*) can treat blood deficiency and insomnia.

本句谚语强调了桂圆米粥对治疗失眠、血虚的药用价值。桂圆，又称龙眼，是生长于我国南方地区的一种水果，具有丰富的营养价值。中医学上认为桂圆味甘、性温，归心、脾经，有开胃、养血益脾、补心安神之功效，因此能够缓解因血虚引起的疲劳、失眠等症。

This proverb emphasizes the medicinal value of rice porridge with dried longan for treating insomnia and blood deficiency. Dried longan is a fruit that is born in southern China. It is rich in nutritional value. In TCM, dried longan tastes sweet and is warm in nature. It enters heart channel and spleen channel, and has the effects of increasing the appetite, nourishing blood and invigorating spleen, and tonifying heart and inducing tranquilization, so it can relieve fatigue and insomnia caused by blood deficiency.

----- 健康小提示 -------------------------------- **Health-preserving Tips**

桂圆属热性食物，一下子不能吃太多。若过食桂圆，会引起上火。孕妇不要多吃，有上火发炎症状的患者不要吃。

Dried longan belongs to hot food, so one can't eat too much at a time. Eating too much dried longan will cause internal fire. Pregnant women should not eat too much dried longan, and patients with inflammation should not eat it.

23 女子不可百日无糖,男子不可百日无姜。

Women can't stay away from [brown] sugar for a long time; men can't stay away from ginger for a long time.

自古以来就有"女子不可百日无糖,男子不可百日无姜"一说。本句谚语强调了男女之间最为简便的补气生血的方法:男子吃姜,女子吃糖。中医学认为生姜味辛,性微温,归肺、脾、胃经,具有解表散寒、温中止呕、温肺止咳的功效;红糖性温,味甘,归肝、脾经,具有益气补血、活血化瘀的作用,对女性极其有益。

Since ancient times, there has been a proverb that goes, "Women can't stay away from [brown] sugar for a long time; men can't stay away from ginger for a long time." This proverb emphasizes the easiest way to replenish *qi* and produce blood between men and women: men should eat ginger and women should eat sugar. In TCM, *shengjiang* (fresh ginger) is pungent in taste, warm in nature, enters the lung channel, spleen channel and stomach channel, and has the effects of releasing the exterior and dispersing cold, warming the middle and stopping vomiting, and warming lung and stopping cough. Brown sugar is warm in nature, sweet in taste, enters the liver channel and spleen channel, and has the functions of nourishing *qi* and blood, and activating blood to dissipate stasis, which is greatly beneficial to women.

----- 健康小提示 ----------------------------- **Health-preserving Tips**

生姜可提升阳气,但不适合在晚上食用,以免造成内火过旺;而秋季时气候干燥,同样不适宜大量食用生姜,以免造成体内失水。

Fresh ginger can increase *yang qi*, but it is not suitable for one to eat at night, so as not to cause internal fire. In autumn, the climate is dry, so it is also not suitable to have large amounts of ginger, so as not to make loss of water in the body.

24 补气补血两大宝,黄芪当归不可少。

Huangqi（milkvetch root）and *danggui*（Chinese angelica）are two treasures to tonify *qi* and blood.

本句谚语强调了黄芪、当归的药用价值,即补气和补血。中医学认为黄芪味甘性温,归肺、脾经,不但可以补全身之气,而且善补肌表之气,尤其对脾气虚所引起的疲倦、乏力、精神萎靡、食欲不振的病患十分有益。当归的主要功效是补血、活血、调经止痛、润燥滑肠。

The proverb emphasizes the medicinal value of *huangqi*（milkvetch root）and *danggui*（Chinese angelica）, namely, tonifying *qi* and blood. In TCM, *huangqi* is sweet in taste and warm in nature, and enters the lung channel and spleen channel. It can not only replenish the *qi* of the whole body, but also replenish the *qi* of the muscles. It is especially beneficial to patients with fatigue, lassitude and loss of appetite caused by spleen-*qi* deficiency. The main effects of *danggui* are to tonify and activate blood, regulate menstruation to relieve pain, and moisten dryness to smooth the intestines.

----- 健康小提示 ---------------------------------- Health-preserving Tips

当归和黄芪在中医学上同属热性药物,因此体质偏热的人不宜食用,否则会内火突旺,危害身体健康。平常人也要适量食用,否则容易上火。

Huangqi and *danggui* are both hot medicines in TCM, so one with hot constitution should not eat them, otherwise the internal heat will increase suddenly, which threatens the health of human body. One should eat them moderately, otherwise it will easily cause internal fire.

25 五谷杂粮壮身体,青菜萝卜保平安。

Coarse grains strengthen human body, and green vegetables and radishes conduce to health.

本句谚语强调了粗粮和蔬菜对维持人体健康的有益之处。通常所说的五谷指的是稻、麦、大豆、玉米、薯类,米、面以外的粮食均称为杂粮。中医学重视饮食均衡,而五谷杂粮种类多,营养齐全,多吃粗粮对补充人体所需的微量元素是极其有益的。而青菜、萝卜含有多种维生素等营养物质,有益于人体健康。

This proverb emphasizes the benefits of coarse grains and vegetables in maintaining human health. Generally speaking, the five cereals refer to rice, wheat, soybeans, corn and tuber crops. Grains other than rice and flour are called miscellaneous grains. TCM attaches great importance to balanced diet, and there are many types of coarse grains with complete nutrition. Eating more coarse grains is extremely beneficial to supply microelements required by human body. Green vegetables and radishes contain a variety of vitamins and other nutrients, which can promote human health.

------ **健康小提示** ---------------------------- **Health-preserving Tips**

吃粗粮的同时应辅以充足的水分,以促进肠道蠕动。

Eating coarse grains should be supplemented with sufficient water to promote intestinal peristalsis.

26　一碗绿豆汤,清热解毒赛仙方。

A bowl of mung bean soup is better than a magic prescription in clearing heat and expelling toxin.

民间常说:"一碗绿豆汤,清热解毒赛仙方。"意思是说喝绿豆汤能够清热下火,排毒润肠,比大夫开的药方都要好。中医学认为,绿豆性寒,归胃经和心经,具有清热、解毒、消暑等功效,尤其适合在夏季食用。

People often say, "A bowl of mung bean soup is better than a magic prescription in clearing heat and expelling toxin." It means that drinking mung bean soup can clear heat, remove the toxin and moisten the intestines, which is better than the prescription provided by doctors. In TCM, mung bean is cold in nature, and enters the stomach channel and heart channel. It has the effects of clearing heat, removing toxin and eliminating summerheat, so it is especially suitable for eating in summer.

------ 健康小提示 ------------------------------ **Health-preserving Tips**

绿豆性寒,因此寒凉体质者不适宜喝。否则会出现全身无力、腰腿冷痛、腹泻等不适之感。同时,中医学上建议不要空腹食用绿豆汤,否则容易伤及脾胃。

Mung bean is cold in nature, so it is not suitable for people with cold constitution. Otherwise, they might incur general weakness, cold waist and leg pain, and diarrhea after drinking. Meanwhile, in TCM, it is not recommended to drink mung bean soup on an empty stomach, which can be prone to damage the stomach and spleen.

27 一碗姜盐茶,开胃祛风寒。

A bowl of salty ginger tea can increase the appetite and dispel the wind-cold.

本句谚语提到了姜盐茶养胃、散风寒的药用功能。姜盐茶由生姜、盐、黄豆、芝麻以及茶叶等共同熬制而成,在民间常用来招待客人。生姜主驱寒发热;食盐可补充人体矿物质;黄豆含有高蛋白质;芝麻性平味甘,具有强身健体之效;而茶叶中含有矿物质和维生素,对人体同样有益。

This proverb mentions the medicinal functions of salty ginger tea to nourish the stomach and dispel wind-cold. Salty ginger tea is made from fresh ginger, salt, soybeans, sesame and tea, and it is commonly used to entertain guests. Ginger can dispel cold and produce heat; salt can supply human minerals; soybeans contain high protein; sesame seeds are sweet in taste and neutral in nature, and have the effect of strengthening the body; tea leaves contain minerals and vitamins, which are also beneficial to human body.

------ 健康小提示 ------------------------------ **Health-preserving Tips**

姜盐茶具有驱寒发汗的作用,因此不宜晚上饮用,饮毕应注意保暖。体质偏热的人群不宜饮用过多。

Salty ginger tea has the effects of dispelling cold and inducing sweat, so it should not be drunk at night. One should keep warm after drinking.

One with hot constitution should not drink too much.

28　木耳抗癌素中荤,姜汤葱辣治感冒。

Wood ear is anti-cancerous and is equal to meat; ginger soup with green onion treats a common cold.

　　我国民间常说:"木耳抗癌素中荤,姜汤葱辣治感冒。"生姜性温,有发汗、解毒的功效,适用于外感风寒;葱味辛,性温,具有发表散寒的功效,对治疗风寒感冒同样有效。而木耳抗癌鲜为人知。中医学认为木耳可以排毒,通脾胃之气,可提高人体免疫力,抵抗疑难杂病。

　　In our country, it is often said that wood ear is anti-cancerous and is equal to meat; ginger soup with green onion treats a common cold. Fresh ginger is warm in nature, has the effects of inducing sweating and removing toxin, and is effective in treating exogenous wind-cold. Green onion is pungent in taste, warm in nature, has the effects of releasing superficies and dispelling cold, and is also effective in treating wind-cold. However, the anti-cancer effect of wood ear is rarely known by people. In TCM, wood ear can remove toxin, free the *qi* in the stomach and spleen, improve human immunity, and resist miscellaneous diseases.

------　健康小提示 -------------------------------- **Health-preserving Tips**

　　干木耳食用前需浸泡,但不要超过8小时. 因为长时间的浸泡会导致木耳被细菌等有害微生物侵袭,最终腐烂变质。人若是吃了这种腐坏的木耳则会食物中毒。

　　Dried wood ear needs to be soaked before eating, but the soaking time should not exceed 8 hours. Because it will be attacked by bacteria and other harmful microorganisms, causing decay and deterioration after a long time of soaking. If one eats this kind of rotten wood ear, there will be food poisoning.

29 马齿苋是个宝,疾病不用尝百草。

Machixian (purslane herb) is a treasure in that it is better than other herbals for treating diseases.

马齿苋是一种植物,产于中国南北各地。性喜肥沃土壤,耐旱亦耐涝,生命力强。马齿苋含有丰富的二羟乙胺、苹果酸、葡萄糖、钙、磷、铁以及维生素等营养物质,既可生食,也可烹饪,能够清除机体内部热毒,还能够消肿止痛,祛湿利尿。因此,民间常谈:"马齿苋是个宝,疾病不用尝百草。"

Machixian (purslane herb) is a plant that is born in many regions of northern and southern China. It favors fertile soil, is tolerant to drought and flood, and has strong vitality. It is rich in nutrients such as dihydroxyethylamine, malic acid, glucose, calcium, phosphorus, iron and vitamins. It can be eaten raw or cooked. It can remove heat toxin from the body, reduce swelling, relieve pain, remove dampness and promote urination. Therefore, people often say, "*Machixian* (purslane herb) is a treasure in that it is better than other herbals for treating diseases."

------ 健康小提示 ----------------------------- **Health-preserving Tips**

夏秋两季,当马齿苋茎叶茂盛时割取全草,洗净泥土,即可药用或食用。

In summer and autumn, it can be harvested with the whole grass when the stems and leaves are luxuriant, and used as medicine or food after washing.

30 生姜拌蜜,咳嗽可医。

Shengjiang (Fresh ginger) mixed with honey can treat cough.

"生姜拌蜜,咳嗽可医"是指用生姜加蜂蜜可治疗风寒咳嗽。一般来说,风寒引起的咳嗽症状有舌色淡、舌苔白,且痰量多、质稀、色白,用生姜拌蜂蜜冲水饮用有疗效。

The proverb "*Shengjiang* (Fresh ginger) mixed with honey can treat cough" refers to the treatment of wind-cold cough through fresh ginger and honey.

Generally speaking, cough caused by wind-cold has the symptoms of pale tongue, white tongue coating, and a lot of sputum with thin quality and white color. So it is better to drink ginger mixed with honey.

------ **健康小提示** --------------------------- **Health-preserving Tips**

风热或燥热引起的咳嗽：舌质红、舌苔黄，且痰量少、质稠、色黄或干咳无痰，此时千万不要用生姜拌蜂蜜，可用蜂蜜炖梨或冰糖煮萝卜水来治疗。当然，如果外感咳嗽久治不愈，且影响脏腑功能而使病变加重，就应抓紧就医，不要再随便用药。

Cough caused by wind-heat or dryness-heat shows red tongue body, yellow tongue coating, low sputum, thick texture, yellow color, or dry cough without phlegm. At this time, do not mix fresh ginger with honey, but stew pears with honey or stew radish with rock candy. Of course, if the exogenous cough can not be cured for a long time, and it affects the function of the viscera and makes the disease worse, one should go to a doctor immediately and stop taking any medicine casually.

31 小儿磨牙，白术可拿。

Baizhu (largehead atractylodes rhizome) can be used for treating bruxism in children.

这则民谚强调了白术对各种原因引起的小儿磨牙具有一定的治疗作用。白术为多年生草本植物。中医认为白术有补脾、益胃、燥湿、和中的功能，以治疗脾胃气虚、不思饮食、倦怠少气、小便不利等证。

This proverb emphasizes that *baizhu* (largehead atractylodes rhizome) has a certain therapeutic effect on bruxism in children caused by various reasons. *Baizhu* is a perennial herb. In TCM, it has the functions of invigorating spleen, replenishing stomach, drying dampness, and harmonizing the middle to treat the symptoms of spleen and stomach *qi* deficiency, loss of appetite, fatigue, shortage of *qi*, and inhibited urination.

----- 健康小提示 ----------------------------- **Health-preserving Tips**

准备适量白术,用温水泡软后放入器皿中,并在上面摊一层蔗糖,然后再加一层白术,如此反复,共用白术100 g,放入笼屉蒸熟。蒸好的白术每次服用15~20 g,可健脾胃。

Prepare some *baizhu*, soak it in warm water and put it in a container, and spread a layer of sucrose on it, and then add a layer of *baizhu* again. Repeat this process, use 100 grams of *baizhu*, and then steam them. Having 15–20 grams of the steamed *baizhu* every time can replenish spleen and stomach.

32 洋葱好味道,防癌抗衰老。

Onion tastes good, prevents cancer and is anti-ageing.

民间有"洋葱好味道,防癌抗衰老"的说法。因为洋葱中含有天然的抗癌物质(栎皮黄素)和抗氧化剂(硒),能提升人体免疫力,防止人体内的细胞变异,并控制癌细胞的生长。人们可以多吃洋葱,强身健体。

There is a saying among folks that "Onion tastes good, prevents cancer and is anti-ageing. " The onion contains natural anti-cancer substances (quercetin) and antioxidants (selenium), which can enhance human immunity, inhibit the growth of cancer cells, prevent cell mutation in human body, and control the growth of cancer cells. People can eat more onions to keep fit.

----- 健康小提示 ----------------------------- **Health-preserving Tips**

洋葱不宜高温烹饪,因为若经高温烹饪,可能产生致癌物质(丙烯酰胺)。所以,日常生活中,生拌洋葱食用即可。

Onions should not be cooked at high temperatures, because carcinogens (acrylamide) may be produced. Therefore, in daily life, one can eat raw onions directly.

33 多吃番茄营养好，貌美年轻疾病少。

Eating more tomatoes keeps one nourished and beautiful, and younger and healthier.

番茄，价格便宜，是人们日常生活中的餐桌常备。中医认为番茄具有健脾消食、生津止渴的作用。番茄中富含维生素 A 和维生素 C，对保护眼睛十分有利。同时，番茄中还含有胡萝卜素和番茄红素，有助于展平皱纹，具有一定的美容护肤功效。

Tomato is cheap, and is common in one's daily life. TCM holds that tomatoes have the functions of invigorating spleen and promoting digestion, and promoting fluid production to quench thirst. Because tomato is rich in vitamin A and vitamin C, it is very beneficial to protect the eyes. At the same time, it also contains carotene and lycopene, which helps to flatten wrinkles and has the effect of beautifying the skin.

----- 健康小提示 ----------------------------- Health-preserving Tips

中医认为番茄属于性寒食物，因此脾胃虚弱者要少吃。女性在经期也不要吃番茄，以免引起痛经。

TCM holds that tomato belongs to a kind of cold food, so one with weak spleen and stomach should eat less, and women should not eat tomatoes during menstruation to avoid dysmenorrhea.

34 石榴止肚痛，简便又易行。

Pomegranate can relieve stomachache, which is simple and easy to achieve.

石榴可用于治疗多种原因引起的腹痛。石榴作为药用非常普遍。其子、叶、花、根都可入药，不过，石榴入药的部位最常用的还要算石榴皮。古今医籍中多有其治疗久泻、久痢、便血、脱肛等病症。如《产经》中治妊娠腹痛的石榴皮汤，即用石榴皮、当归、阿胶、艾叶四味药共同煎汤。

Pomegranate can be used to treat abdominal pain caused by many reasons. It is very popular for medicinal purposes. Its seeds, leaves, flowers, and roots can be used as medicine, but the most commonly used part of pomegranate as medicine is pomegranate peel. In ancient and modern medical books, it has been used to treat chronic diarrhea, chronic dysentery, blood in the stool, rectal prolapse, and other diseases. For example, in the book *Chan Jing* (*Records of Gynaecological and Paediatric Diseases*), the pomegranate peel soup is used to treat abdominal pain during pregnancy. It is decocted with four herbs: peel of pomegranate, *danggui* (Chinese angelica), *ejiao* (ass hide glue), and *aiye* (argy wormwood leaf).

----- 健康小提示 ----------------------------- **Health-preserving Tips**

日常生活中可以吃一些石榴,因为石榴确实可以治疗腹痛腹泻,石榴里面含有鞣酸、维生素 C、柠檬酸、苹果酸等,有助于消化。

One can eat some pomegranate, because it indeed treats abdominal pain and diarrhea. It contains tannic acid, vitamin C, citric acid, malic acid, etc. , which are helpful for digestion.

35 多吃五谷杂粮,少生疮疡杂病。
Eat coarse grains more, get sick less.

民间常说:"多吃五谷杂粮,少生疮疡杂病。"这则谚语强调了平常多吃五谷杂粮有益身体健康。五谷杂粮包含多种粮食作物,不同的粮食含有不同的营养物质。因此,多吃混合粮食作物能够保证机体对营养的全面需要。

Folks often say, "Eat coarse grains more, get sick less. " This proverb emphasizes that eating more coarse grains is good for human health. Coarse grains contain a variety of food crops, and different foods contain different nutrients. Therefore, eating more mixed crops can ensure human body's overall nutritional needs.

----- 健康小提示 ----------------------------- **Health-preserving Tips**

在日常生活中要多吃一些五谷杂粮,比如豆类、稻谷、小麦。

In daily life, one should eat more coarse grains, such as beans, rice, and wheat.

36　冬瓜消肿又利尿,清热减肥抗衰老。

Chinese waxgourd induces diuresis, alleviates edema, clears heat, loses weight, and resists aging.

本句谚语强调了冬瓜的保健作用。中医认为冬瓜性寒味甘,有清热生津、祛湿解暑、消炎降火的功效。同时,冬瓜不含脂肪,热量十分低,所以是减肥期间很好的食品。体重不理想的人群可以通过食用冬瓜来达到减肥清脂的目的。

This proverb emphasizes the health benefits of Chinese waxgourd. TCM holds that Chinese waxgourd is cold in nature and sweet in taste, and has the effects of clearing heat and promoting fluid production, dispelling dampness and clearing summerheat, eliminating inflammation to reduce fire. At the same time, Chinese waxgourd does not contain fat, and is also very low in calories, so it is a good choice during weight loss. For one with unsatisfactory weight, he/she can eat Chinese waxgourd to achieve the goal of weight loss and fat removal.

------ 健康小提示 ------------------------------------ **Health-preserving Tips**

冬瓜性寒,所以脾胃气虚者、胃寒疼痛者忌食生冬瓜,月经期间的女性也要忌食生冬瓜。

Chinese waxgourd is cold in nature, so one with deficiency of spleen and stomach *qi* and stomach cold should not eat raw waxgourd, and women during menstruation should also avoid eating it.

37　香蕉润肠通便好,降压解郁抗疲劳。

Banana is good to moisten intestines to relieve constipation, release pressure to relieve depression, and resist fatigue.

香蕉是一种十分常见的水果。香蕉富含钾元素,有辅助降低血压的功效;同时,其中所含的一种能够帮助人体产生羟色胺的物质,能使人的心情变得愉悦,减轻忧郁;香蕉所含的食物纤维,可以刺激大肠的蠕动,使大便通畅,因此可以防治习惯性便秘。因此,民间常说"香蕉润肠通便好,降压解郁抗疲劳"。

Banana is a very common fruit. Banana is rich in potassium, which can help lower blood pressure. Meanwhile, it contains a substance that can help the body produce serotonin, which can make people feel happy and relieve depression. The dietary fiber contained in the banana can stimulate large intestines to move and relax the bowels, so it can prevent habitual constipation. Therefore, people often say, "Banana is good to moisten intestines to relieve constipation, release pressure to relieve depression, and resist fatigue."

----- **健康小提示** ----------------------------------- **Health-preserving Tips**

香蕉中含有大量的糖分和钾,每天吃1~2根就足够了。因为香蕉性寒,所以高血糖人群,虚寒、胃痛、腹泻的人要少吃。

Banana contains a lot of sugar and potassium, so one should not eat more than one or two bananas every day. Banana is cold in nature, so one with high blood sugar, deficiency of cold, stomachache, and diarrhea should eat less.

38 甘蔗甜又甜,清热又消炎。
Sugarcane is sweet, which can clear heat and eliminate inflammation.

想到甘蔗,口中立即会有甜蜜的滋味。甘蔗会让人联想到甜,尤其是在炎热的夏季,喝上一口冰镇的甘蔗汁非常舒爽。因为甘蔗水分充足,而且性凉,所以可治疗肺热咳嗽、气喘痰多、口干咽燥等症状。

There will be sweet in the one's mouth immediately at the thought of sugarcane. Sugarcane will make one think of sweetness. Especially in the hot summer, it is very comfortable and relaxed for one to drink a sip of iced sugarcane juice. Because sugarcane has sufficient water and is cold in nature, it can treat lung heat, cough, wheezing, excessive phlegm, dry mouth and throat.

----- **健康小提示** ----------------------------------- **Health-preserving Tips**

蔗汁性凉,虚寒体质人员不适合多饮,若寒咳(痰白而稀)者误饮,病况有可

能即时加剧。

Sugarcane juice is cold in nature, so one with deficiency-cold constitution had better not drink more. If one with cold cough (white and thin sputum) drinks by mistake, the disease may get worse immediately.

39　柑橘营养价值高,理气健脾润秋燥。

Citrus has high nutritional value, which regulates *qi* and invigorates spleen, and moistens autumn-dryness.

柑橘资源丰富,种类繁多,人们生活中常见的橘子、柚子、橙子、柠檬等都属于柑橘类水果。柑橘营养丰富,民间常说"柑橘营养价值高,理气健脾润秋燥"。以橘子为例,中医认为橘子全身都是宝。比如橘皮含有大量的维生素 C,具有理气化痰,健脾胃的作用;橘络可以保护血管,可以直接吃,也可以用来泡水喝;橘核可理气、散结。

Citrus has rich resources and various varieties. Tangerines, grapefruit, oranges and lemons, which are common in people's life, belong to citrus fruits. Citrus has high nutritional value. It is often said that citrus has high nutritional value, which regulates *qi* and invigorates spleen, and moistens autumn-dryness. Taking tangerines as an example, TCM holds that tangerines are a total treasure. For example, tangerine peel contains a large amount of vitamin C, which has the effects of regulating *qi* and resolving phlegm, invigorating spleen and stomach; tangerine collaterals can protect blood vessels and can be eaten directly or soaked; tangerine nuclei can regulate *qi* and dissipate nodulation.

------ 健康小提示 ----------------------------- **Health-preserving Tips**

柑橘类水果中,柚子可以去体内火气,橙子比较温和,而其他都易导致上火。因此,体质偏热的人群要少吃柑橘类水果。

Among citrus fruits, grapefruit can remove the heat in human body; oranges are mild in nature, while others are easy to cause inner heat. Therefore, one with hot constitution should eat less citrus fruits.

40 多吃小辣椒，寿数节节高。

Eating more chili and enjoying longer life.

这则谚语强调了吃辣椒的好处。我国许多地方都有长期吃辣椒的习惯，比如四川、贵州、湖南等地。辣椒不仅是一种美味的食材，更是一味保健中药。中医认为，辣椒味辛，性温中，可以驱寒，对于缓解胃寒疼痛，排胃气，治疗消化不良、冻疮等有一定帮助。

This proverb emphasizes the benefits of eating chili. Many places in our country have the habit of eating chili, such as Sichuan, Guizhou, Hunan and other provinces. Chili is not only a delicious food, but also a Chinese drug for health preservation. TCM holds that chili is pungent in taste and warm in nature, which can dispel cold. It is helpful to relieve stomach-cold and stomach-pain, discharge stomach qi, and treat indigestion and frostbite.

------ 健康小提示 ------------------------------ Health-preserving Tips

辣椒摄入过量可能会对口腔和胃黏膜产生刺激，因此不建议本身脾胃虚弱的人群食用。

Excessive chili may cause irritation to the oral cavity and gastric mucosa, so it is not recommended for one with weak stomach and spleen to eat it.

第三节　饮食禁忌
Section Three　Food Prohibition

1 天时虽热，不可食凉。

Although the weather is hot, do not eat something cold.

民间常说："天时虽热，不可食凉。"暗示吃凉东西会对身体造成危害，尤其是在暑天。中医认为，夏天人的阳气往外走，身体内部是寒的，一旦吃过多的凉东西,肠胃会受凉,蠕动能力减弱,影响人体的吸收功能。

People often say, "Although the weather is hot, do not eat something cold." The proverb implies that eating something cold will cause harm to the body, especially in summer. TCM holds that in summer, *yang qi* of human body goes out and the exterior of human body is cold. Once eating too much cold food, the stomach and intestines will be cold and the peristaltic ability will be weakened, which will affect the body's absorption function.

----- 健康小提示 ------------------------------ **Health-preserving Tips**

夏天天气炎热,人们都喜爱吃冷饮,但需注意,生吃瓜果和冷饮要适量,因为过量食用生冷的东西,会导致脾胃不适,出现胃痛、腹痛、腹泻等症状,尤其是有胃病的人更应少吃或不吃。

People like to have cold drinks in summer. But having raw melons and fruits and cold drinks should be moderated, because overeating will cause the discomfort of stomach and spleen, stomach pain, abdominal pain and diarrhea, especially for people with stomach problems.

2 吃饭不要闹,吃饱不要跳。
No frolicing during a meal, no running after a meal.

人们常说:"吃饭不要闹,吃饱不要跳。"说明吃饭的时候不应嬉戏打闹,而饭后不应剧烈运动。吃饭时打闹不仅是一种不良生活习惯,还直接分散人的注意力,影响进食规律,容易导致消化不良。饭后指的是吃饭后不久的那段时间,因为这段时间刚刚吃完饭,肚子里面的食物还没有消化好,所以饭后不应该剧烈运动。

People often say, "No frolicing during a meal, no running after a meal." It means that one should keep quiet when eating, and should not take exercise vigorously after eating. Romping while eating is not only a bad life habit, but also directly distracts one's attention, affects dietary rules, and easily leads to indigestion. "After a meal" refers to a short period after eating. Because the food in the stomach has not been digested just after the meal, one should not take exercise vigorously after a meal.

饭后一个小时左右进行运动,效果最好,尤其是对于一些消化不良的患者,有助于消化,对于其身体的营养吸收也有好处。

Taking exercises an hour after a meal has the best effect, especially for some patients with indigestion, which is good for digestion and nutrient absorption of the body.

3　五味不衡,百病丛生。

[If] the five flavors are not balanced, people will suffer from various diseases.

中医将食物大致分为五味:酸、苦、甘、辛和咸。俗话说:"五味不衡,百病丛生。"这则谚语提示我们饮食五味要均衡。《黄帝内经》中就描述五味不衡对身体造成的不同危害:多食咸,则脉凝泣而变色;多食苦,则皮槁而毛拔;多食辛,则筋急而爪枯;多食酸,则肉胝而唇揭;多食甘,则骨痛而发落。

In TCM, food can be divided according to five flavors: sour, bitter, sweet, pungent and salty. As the saying goes, "[If] the five flavors are not balanced, people will suffer from various diseases." This proverb reminds us to have a balanced diet with five flavors. *Huang Di Nei Jing* (*Huangdi's Canon of Medicine*) mentions the harm to human body by imbalanced five flavors: Excessive taking of salty food stagnates the blood vessels and changes the countenance. Excessive taking of bitter food makes the skin dry and body hair lose. Excessive taking of pungent food causes cramp of musculature and dry nails. Excessive taking of sour food leads to wrinkled thickness of the muscles and chap of the lips. Excessive taking of sweet food results in pain of bones and loss of hair.

五味均衡的原则:其一,食物不过咸;其二,食物不过甜;其三,食物不过腻(限制脂肪过高的食品);其四,食物不过辛;其五,食物不过苦。

The principles of five-flavor balance are: Firstly, food should not be too salty; secondly, food should not be too sweet; thirdly, food should not be too greasy (high fat); fourthly, food should not be too spicy; fifthly, food should not be too bitter.

4　莫吃空心茶, 少食中夜饭。

Do not drink on an empty stomach; do not eat at night.

《类修要诀》中说: "莫吃空心茶, 少食中夜饭", 说明了空腹吃喝的害处。空腹饮茶会稀释胃液, 降低消化功能, 容易引起胃炎。夜间本是该休息的时间, 如果经常进食会导致身体机能紊乱, 胃部鼓胀, 压迫周围器官, 进而影响身体健康。

There is a saying in the book *Lei Xiu Yao Jue* (*Key to Preserving Health*) that goes, "Do not drink on an empty stomach; do not eat at night." This indicates that it is harmful to eat or drink on an empty stomach. Drinking tea on an empty stomach will dilute gastric juice, weaken digestive function, and easily cause gastritis. At night, it is the time for rest. Eating at night often will cause disorders of body functions, swelling of the stomach, pressure on surrounding organs, and thus threatening the health.

------ 健康小提示 -------------------------- **Health-preserving Tips**

空腹和饭前不宜饮茶。因为茶水会冲淡唾液, 使饮食无味, 还会导致消化器官吸收蛋白质的功能下降。

It is not suitable to drink tea on an empty stomach or before meals because it will dilute saliva, make the food tasteless, and also weaken the function of digestive organs for absorbing protein.

5　肥腻伤体, 甜食坏身。

Greasy food and sweetmeat hurt human body.

"肥腻伤体, 甜食坏身"这句谚语强调了高脂肪类食物和高糖分类食物对人体健康的危害。中医认为肥甘厚味酿湿生痰, 容易导致肥胖。而各类甜食的主

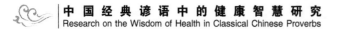

要成分就是糖。糖本身并无危害,但摄入过多会导致骨质疏松、营养不良、发胖以及糖尿病等。因此,少吃高脂高糖类食品,尤其是中老年人,对维持身体健康十分重要。

The proverb "Greasy food and sweetmeat hurt human body" emphasizes the harm to human health from high-fat foods and high-sugar foods. TCM holds that high-fat foods and high-sugar foods cause dampness and phlegm, and easily lead to obesity. The main ingredient of all kinds of sweets is sugar. Sugar itself is not harmful, but too much intake of it can lead to osteoporosis, malnutrition, obesity and diabetes. Therefore, eating less high-fat and high-sugar foods is very important for keeping healthy especially for middle-aged and elderly people.

------ **健康小提示** ----------------------------------- **Health-preserving Tips**

为了肠胃的健康,饮食应以清淡为主,建议多吃蔬菜、豆类、水果、谷物和坚果。

In order to keep intestines and stomach healthy, one's diet should be light. And it is recommended to eat more vegetables, beans, fruits, grains and nuts.

6 生吃螃蟹活吃虾,健康远离病至家。

[If one] eats raw crabs and shrimps, health will be reachless and diseases will be unavoidable.

该句谚语强调了吃生冷食物的危害。民间常流传着一句话:"生吃螃蟹活吃虾,健康远离病至家。"部分地区的人有生吃螃蟹和虾的习惯,因为他们认为这样可以长力气。但是生的食物中很可能会有寄生虫卵,尤其是海鲜产品,如果生吃就会导致寄生虫感染,从而引起一些疾病,所以在吃海鲜的时候需要做熟再吃。

This proverb emphasizes the dangers of eating raw or cold food. There is often a saying among the folks, "[If one] eat raw crabs and shrimps, health will be reachless and diseases will be unavoidable." People in some areas have the habit of eating raw crabs and shrimps because they think they can strengthen power. However, there may be parasite eggs in raw food, especially in seafood products.

Eating something raw will cause parasite infection and then cause other diseases. Therefore, one should cook seafood before eating.

------ **健康小提示** ---------------------------- **Health-preserving Tips**

吃海鲜时不宜畅饮啤酒,否则容易导致血尿酸水平急剧升高,诱发痛风,以致出现痛风性肾病、痛风性关节炎等。

It is not advisable to drink beer while eating seafood, otherwise there might be a sharp increase in blood uric acid level and gout, resulting in gouty nephropathy and gouty arthritis.

7　鱼生火,肉生痰,粗粮淡茶保平安。
Fish produces fire, meat causes phlegm, but coarse food grain and weak tea keep people in good health.

民间有俗语"鱼生火,肉生痰,粗粮淡茶保平安",强调了鱼和肉虽好,但不宜过量,还是粗粮有益身体健康。中医认为鱼属于温性食物,吃多了会导致内火过旺,所以称之为"鱼生火"。肉类含有大量的脂肪,摄入过多的话,会导致体内津液代谢失常,产生痰浊现象。当然只要适量食用,鱼和肉不会带来"生火"和"生痰"的问题。

A folk saying goes that "Fish produces fire, meat causes phlegm, but coarse food grain and weak tea keep people in good health." It emphasizes that although fish and meat are good, they should not be over eaten. In fact, coarse grains are good for health. TCM holds that fish belongs to warm food, and eating too much will cause excessive internal fire, so people believe that "fish produces fire". There is a lot of fat in meat. If people eat too much, it will cause abnormal body fluid metabolism and phlegm turbidity. Of course, as long as people eat them in moderation, the problems of causing fire and phlegm will not arise.

------ **健康小提示** ---------------------------- **Health-preserving Tips**

生活中不可一味追求大鱼大肉以及精米、精面等食品,应当多吃一些粗粮和蔬菜,比如玉米、红薯、萝卜和各种青菜等,这样有利于保持营养均衡、促进身体健康。

One in daily life should not always eat too much fish or meat, refined rice or noodles, etc. One should eat more coarse grains and vegetables, such as corn, sweet potatoes, radishes and various green vegetables. These contribute to balanced nutrition and promote physical fitness.

8 怒后不可便食，食后不可发怒。

Do not eat after getting angry; do not get angry after having food.

清代卓有成就的学者和文学家梁章钜曾说："怒后不可便食，食后不可发怒。"生活中经常有人在生气发怒的时候没有胃口，吃不下饭，其实这是因为肝气郁结所致。中医认为人体五脏之间互相关联，而生气会造成肝气郁结，进而影响脾胃，导致消化功能减退。

Liang Zhangju, an accomplished scholar and writer in the Qing Dynasty, once said, "Do not eat after getting angry; do not get angry after having food." One often has no appetite when he/she is angry. In fact, this is caused by stagnation of liver *qi*. TCM holds that the five *zang* viscera of human body are related to each other, and anger can cause stagnation of liver *qi*, which in turn affects the stomach and spleen, leading to poor digestive function.

------ 健康小提示 ----------------------------- **Health-preserving Tips**

学着调节个人情绪，生气的时候不要进食，进食后也不要发怒。尤其是肝火旺的人要注意保持心情舒畅。因此，一般人日常可以吃苦瓜来降火。

One should learn to adjust emotions. One should not eat when he/she gets angry, and should not get angry after having food. Especially one with exuberant liver fire should stay in a good mood. One can eat bitter gourd to reduce inner heat in daily life.

9 饱食即卧，乃生百病。

Lying down immediately after meal will cause diseases.

唐代医药学家孙思邈在其所著《备急千金要方》中提到："饱食即卧，乃生百病。"吃饱了就睡,食物停留在胃中无法得以消化,会导致积食,损伤脾胃,气血痰食积聚而致百病丛生。

Sun Simiao mentioned in his book *Bei Ji Qian Jin Yao Fang* (*Golden Prescriptions for Emergency Use*), "Lying down immediately after meal will cause diseases." Going to sleep after meal is not good. At this time, food stays in the stomach and cannot be digested. This will cause food accumulation, damage the spleen and stomach, and accumulate *qi*, blood, sputum and food, which eventually cause diseases.

----- 健康小提示 ----------------------------- **Health-preserving Tips**

好的健康习惯就是吃饭之后进行适当的轻微运动,比如散步,可以促进食物的消化吸收。

It is a good habit to take some exercise after eating, such as walking, which can promote the digestion and absorption of food.

10　吃得慌,咽得忙,伤了胃口害了肠。

Eating and swallowing in a hurry do harm to the appetite and the intestines.

中国人至古以来都讲究细嚼慢咽,认为狼吞虎咽的吃饭方式不仅有碍观瞻,对身体健康也不好。所以民间常说"吃得慌,咽得忙,伤了胃口害了肠",强调吃饭过快对身体有害。中医上认为吃饭太快会导致消化不良,因为进食速度过快,胃部的消化液无法及时分泌出来,所以会导致食物在胃部堆积,造成不消化的现象。

Since ancient times, Chinese people have always valued chewing and eating slowly. It is believed that the way of eating gluttonously not only does not follow the table manners, but also does harm to health. Therefore, people often say "Eating and swallowing in a hurry do harm to the appetite and the intestines", emphasizing that eating too fast is harmful to the body. In TCM, eating too fast will cause indigestion. Because the digestive juice of human stomach cannot be secreted in time, which will cause food to accumulate in the stomach and lead to indigestion.

------ 健康小提示 ------------------------------ **Health-preserving Tips**

日常吃饭要预留出时间,不要摄取过多,也不要吃过快,更不要为了赶工作而忽略一日三餐,这样才能预防各种疾病。

One should set aside time for daily meals, and should not eat too much, eat too fast, or even neglect meals because of busy affairs. Only in this way, various diseases may be prevented.

11 桃养人,杏伤人,李子树下埋死人。

Peach nourishes human body; apricot hurts human body; the dead are buried under the plum tree.

这则谚语说明了三种水果的不同特点。从字面来看,多吃桃子有助于人的身体健康,吃太多杏会危害人体健康,而吃多了李子可能会致人死亡,所以也就有了"李子树下埋死人"这一说法。中医上,桃性温,味甘酸,具有补气养血、养阴生津的功效;杏微温,甘酸,有微毒,多食易生痰和热;与杏一样,李子吃多了也会生痰,多食会中毒。

This proverb explains the different characteristics of the three fruits. Literally, eating more peaches is helpful to one's health. Eating too many apricots is harmful to human health. And eating too many plums may cause death, that's why there is a saying that the dead are buried under the plum tree. In TCM, peaches are warm in nature, sweet and sour in taste, and have the effects of tonifying *qi* and nourishing blood, nourishing *yin* and promoting fluid production; apricots are mildly warm in nature, sweet and sour in taste, and are slightly toxic. Eating too many will cause phlegm and heat. Like apricots, eating too many plums will also cause phlegm and lead to food poisoning.

------ 健康小提示 ------------------------------ **Health-preserving Tips**

中医上认为饮食需有节。不论是桃子、杏子还是李子,本身都没有什么坏处,但如果吃太多的话,反而会造成一些伤害。

TCM believes that diet should be moderate. Peaches, apricots or plums, are not harmful, but too much taking at one time will do harm to the body.

12　宁尝鲜桃一口,不吃烂杏一筐。

[I] would rather eat a mouthful of fresh peaches than eat a basket of rotten apricots.

本句谚语采用了比喻的修辞手法,意思是说宁愿吃少量新鲜的食物,也不愿意吃变质的食物。这个道理很简单,不管是饭菜、水果还是肉类,一旦变质都会滋生大量有害人体健康的细菌,所以应吃新鲜的食物。

This proverb uses a metaphor, which means that one would rather eat a small amount of fresh food than spoiled food. The reason is very simple. Whether it is food, fruit or meat, once it is spoiled, it will breed a large number of harmful bacteria, so food should be eaten fresh.

------- 健康小提示 ------------------------------- **Health-preserving Tips**

在生活中,我们应选择合理的方式储存食物。现代家庭普遍使用冰箱等冷藏机,需注意储存水果蔬菜的保鲜冷库温度范围一般在0℃~15℃。

In daily life, one should select correct ways of storing different foods. Refrigerators are commonly used in modern family. It should be noted that the temperature range of storing fruit and vegetables is generally between 0℃ and 15℃.

13　大饥而食宜软,大渴而饮宜温。

[One should] eat soft food when being very hungry; [one should] drink warm water when being very thirsty.

这则谚语说明非常饿的时候,要吃软食;非常渴的时候,要喝温水。极度饥饿的状态下,人的肠道会变得非常脆弱,若进食硬的食物,容易造成消化不良、肠道出血。而极度口渴时突然喝凉水易造成肠胃功能紊乱。同时,中医认为饮用温水可以温煦阳气,有利于胃中已腐食物的消化,更有利于脾胃的消化吸收和新陈代谢。

This proverb states that when one is very hungry, he/she should eat something soft, and when one is very thirsty, he/she should drink something warm. For a starving person, his/her intestines become very fragile. If one eats hard food, it is easy to cause indigestion and intestinal bleeding. Drinking cold water suddenly when one is extremely thirsty is easy to cause gastrointestinal disorders. At the same time, TCM holds that drinking warm water can warm *yang qi*, which is helpful for the digestion of rotten food in the stomach, and is more conducive to the digestion, absorption and metabolism of the spleen and the stomach.

----- **健康小提示** ------------------------------ **Health-preserving Tips**

长久饥饿之下,切莫狼吞虎咽生硬之物;酷热口渴之下,切莫饮用冰凉的水。

Under the condition of long-term hunger, one should not swallow hard things; under the condition of severe heat and thirst, one should not drink cold water.

14 饭菜嚼成浆,身体必健康。
Chew the food into pulp is conducive to health.

这则谚语同样是强调吃饭时细嚼慢咽对身体有好处。经过细嚼的食物,能扩大与肠壁的接触面积,消化也能够充分发挥作用,从而使肠壁广泛地吸收食物中的养分。此外,细嚼慢咽还可以提前促进胃液和其他消化腺分泌增多,为食物进入胃肠后充分被吸收做好准备,从而减轻胃的负担。

This proverb also emphasizes that eating slowly is good for human body. By chewing food, the contact area with the intestinal wall is expanded, and digestive function takes great effect, so that the intestinal wall can absorb nutrients from food widely. In addition, chewing and swallowing slowly can also increase the secretion of gastric juice and other digestive glands in advance, and prepare for full absorption of food after entering the gastrointestinal tract, thereby reducing the burden on the stomach.

----- **健康小提示** ------------------------------ **Health-preserving Tips**

吃东西时要有意识地反复咀嚼食物,给口腔足够的时间来分泌唾液,这样不

但有助于消食,还能起到杀菌的作用,预防牙部疾病。

One should chew food repeatedly so as to allow enough time for the oral cavity to secrete saliva, which not only promotes the digestion of food, but also has a sterilization effect and prevents dental diseases.

15　甜言夺志,甜食坏齿。

Sweet words kill ambition; sweet food hurts teeth.

民间有句谚语说得好:"甜言夺志,甜食坏齿。"在中医理论中,甜入脾走肉,脾属土,主运化,而土克水,肾属水,因此甜食坏齿。当然,甜食在牙齿上黏着,会滋生细菌,细菌将甜食消化利用,生成腐蚀牙齿的酸,进而也会影响牙齿。

As the proverb goes, "Sweet words kill ambition; sweet food hurts teeth." In the theory of TCM, sweetness enters the spleen channel and the muscles. The spleen belongs to soil and governs transportation and transformation, while the soil restrains water, so sweet food spoils the teeth. Furthermore, the sticking of sweets on the teeth will breed bacteria. The bacteria will digest and use the sweets to generate acid that corrodes and destroys the teeth.

----- 健康小提示 ----------------------------- **Health-preserving Tips**

人们应多吃低糖食物,比如喝脱脂牛奶、低糖牛奶、酸奶。老年人吃糖的时候应多吃红糖或黑糖。

People should eat low-sugar foods more, such as skimmed milk, low-sugar milk or yogurt. The elderly should choose brown sugar when eating sugar.

16　人愿长寿安,要减夜来餐。

If people want to live a long and peaceful life, they need to eat less at night.

自古以来,我国就有"人愿长寿安,要减夜来餐"一说,强调了夜晚吃东西的危害,主要是为了规劝大家不要吃夜宵。

Since ancient times, there has been a saying in our country that goes, "If people want to live a long and peaceful life, they need to eat less at night." It indicates the harm of eating something at night, and is mainly to persuade people not to eat night snacks.

----- 健康小提示 ------------------------------- **Health-preserving Tips**

傍晚6点左右进晚餐较合适，因为人的排钙高峰期常在进餐后4~5小时，若晚餐过晚，会错过排钙高峰期，毒素就会滞留体内，危害健康。

One should have dinner at around 6 o'clock in the evening, because the peak period of calcium excretion will come 4—5 hours after eating. If one eats too late, the peak period of calcium excretion will be missed. The toxin cannot be discharged in time, staying in the body and threatening health.

17 热饭不能热食。

The meal can not be eaten when it is hot.

常言道："热饭不能热食"，说的是烫嘴的饭吃下去会对肠胃有害，因此不能吃。这同样强调了为人做事不能操之过急，要有耐心。太热的饭，容易损伤胃黏膜和食道黏膜，长此以往，易引发病变乃至癌症。胃不好的人，吃饭更应注意要冷热适度。

As the saying goes, "The meal can not be eaten when it is hot." It means that too hot food is harmful to the stomach and intestines, so one should not eat. This also emphasizes that one can't do things in haste, and should be patient. Too hot food tends to damage the gastric mucosa and esophageal mucosa. Long-term damage to the stomach and esophageal mucosa will easily cause cancer. One with a bad stomach should pay more attention to take in food with moderate temperature.

----- 健康小提示 ------------------------------- **Health-preserving Tips**

人们应养成良好的生活习惯，多饮水，忌食生冷和辛辣的东西。饭菜温度须适中，过冷过热皆会损伤脾胃。

It is recommended that one should develop good living habits: drink plenty of water and avoid eating something cold and spicy. The meal should be in moderate temperature. Food that is too cold or too hot is harmful to spleen and stomach.

18　荤素搭配，精神百倍。

A balanced diet of meat and vegetables is good for health.

　　这则谚语强调了饮食要合理，不能偏食。"荤"和"素"是一对相对的概念。"荤"常指肉蛋类食物，而"素"则指蔬菜和粮食。吃素的好处不用多说。吃荤能提高人体蛋白质和脂肪的含量，为身体提供充足的热量，但吃荤太多会引发心血管疾病等，不足则难以维持身体热能所需。所以，吃荤吃素要均衡。

　　This proverb emphasizes that the diet should be rationally balanced. "Hun" and "Su" are a pair of relative concepts. "Hun" usually refers to meat and eggs, while "Su" refers to vegetables and grains. There is no need to talk about the benefits of eating "Su". Eating meat and eggs can increase the content of human body's protein and fat and provide sufficient energy for human body. However, eating too much meat will cause cardiovascular disease, etc., and if not enough, it will be difficult to maintain human body's heat energy needs. Therefore, eating meat and vegetables should be balanced.

------ 健康小提示 ---------------------------- **Health-preserving Tips**

　　饮食不应偏食，每天的肉食和素食都应合理搭配，均衡饮食，不能偏于一方。

The diet should be balanced. People should take in meat and vegetables every day in a reasonable manner. It is inadvisable to eat meat or vegetables only in daily diets.

19　油多菜香，一哄而光。

The dish with much oil smells delicious and is eaten up in no time.

　　民谚有云："油多菜香，一哄而光。"在中国，油是人们生活中的主要调味品，人们炒菜必定少不了油。油用来炒菜虽香，但也不是吃得越多越好。油中含有大量脂肪，食用过多易导致肥胖，引发高血压、心血管疾病等。

There is a proverb that goes, "The dish with much oil smells delicious and is eaten up in no time." In China, oil is the main condiment in people's lives, and it is indispensable for people to cook. Although oil is fragrant when used for cooking, eating more is not always better. Oil contains a lot of fat. Having too much leads to obesity, high blood pressure and cardiovascular diseases.

----- 健康小提示 ---------------------------- **Health-preserving Tips**

油是调味品,不宜吃太多,尤其对中老年人来说,饮食应以清淡为主,且应多吃一些植物油。

Oil is a condiment and should not be eaten too much. Middle-aged and elderly people, especially should keep the diet light and eat more vegetable oil.

20　李子止渴又生津,多食反而会伤身。
Plum promotes fluid-production to quench thirst, but overeating hurts human body.

李子,又名嘉庆子,在我国很多地方都有种植。李子味甘酸,性平,入肝、肾两经,具有清热、生津、利水、健胃的功效。因此,人们常说"李子生津又止渴"。但又有"桃养人,杏伤人,李子树下埋死人"的说法,实则是在强调过食李子的危害之大。李子酸含量高,吃太多容易伤脾胃,引起腹胀等现象。

Plums, also known as *jia qing zi*, are grown in many places in China. Plum is sweet and sour in taste and neutral in nature, enters the liver channel and kidney channel, and has the effects of clearing heat, promoting fluid production, inducing diuresis, and invigorating stomach. Therefore, it is often said that plum promotes fluid-production to quench thirst, but overeating hurts human body. However, there is a saying that "Peaches nourish people, apricots hurt people, and dead people are buried under plum trees", which actually has emphasized the great harm of overeating plums. Because of the high acid content of plums, eating too much can easily hurt stomach and spleen and cause abdominal distension.

----- 健康小提示 ---------------------------- **Health-preserving Tips**

肠胃消化不良者应少吃李子,否则会引起轻微的腹泻。而多食李子会使人

生痰、助湿,甚至令人发虚热,所以脾胃虚弱者也应少吃。

One with gastrointestinal indigestion should eat less plums, otherwise it will cause mild diarrhea. Overeating causes phlegm and even heat-deficiency, so one with weak stomach and spleen should also eat less.

21　忌吃未煮熟的四季豆,不吃发了芽的马铃薯。

One should never eat half-cooked kidney beans and sprouted potatoes.

四季豆和马铃薯(土豆)是人们常吃的蔬菜,但民间常说"忌吃未煮熟的四季豆,不吃发了芽的马铃薯"。因为四季豆本身含有毒蛋白(溶血素和凝集素),只有在高温下才能被破坏,所以当人们食用了加热温度不够的豆角时,就会出现恶心、头晕的现象。马铃薯也同样如此,本身含有天然毒素,若食用过多或吃了发芽的,可能会导致急性中毒。

Kidney beans and potatoes are vegetables that people often eat. A proverb goes that "One should never eat half-cooked kidney beans and sprouted potatoes." Because kidney beans contain toxic proteins (hemolysin and lectins) that can only be destroyed at high temperature. Therefore, when people eat beans that are not cooked enough, they will suffer from nausea and dizziness. The same is true of potatoes. They contain natural toxins. If people eat too many or sprouted potatoes, they may suffer from acute poisoning.

------ 健康小提示 ----------------------------- **Health-preserving Tips**

家中煸炒四季豆和马铃薯时应高温烹饪,尤其是发芽的马铃薯,应弃之不食。

Stir-frying kidney beans and potatoes at home should be performed at high temperature. Germinated potatoes should be discarded immediately.

第三章 健康谚语运动篇

Chapter Three Health-preserving Proverbs About Exercise

第一节 形神俱养

Section One Nourishing Physique and *Shen*（spirit）Together

1 精神不运则愚,血脉不运则病。

The unused brain makes one foolish, and the obstructed vessels make one sick.

南宋哲学家陆九渊在《象山语录》中说:"精神不运则愚,血脉不运则病。"大脑越用越灵活,气血通畅对人体健康大有裨益。

"The unused brain makes one foolish, and the obstructed vessels make one sick," Lu Jiuyuan, a philosopher of the Southern Song Dynasty, said in *Xiang Shan Yu Lu*（*Important words spoken in Xiang Mountain*）. The more the brain is used, the more flexible it becomes. Unobstructed *qi* and blood are of great benefit to human health.

----- 健康小提示 -------------------------------- **Health-preserving Tips**

平时多阅读,可以提升大脑的创造力和想象力。另外,坚持体育锻炼,有助于人体气血通畅。

Reading more can improve the creativity and imagination of the brain. In addition, insisting on physical exercise is helpful to the smooth flow of *qi* and blood.

2　百忧感其心,万事劳其形。

Endless worries torment one's mood, and countless trifles exhaust one's body.

北宋文学家欧阳修在古典散文《闲居赋·秋声赋》中说:"百忧感其心,万事劳其形。"中医学认为心对整个人体生命活动起着主宰的作用,因此被称为"君主之官"。令人不快的这些事情很容易便会损伤人的心神。

"Endless worries torment one's mood, and countless trifles exhaust one's body," Ouyang Xiu, a litterateur of the Northern Song Dynasty, said in *Qiu Sheng Fu* (*Odes to the Sound of Autumn & Living in Idleness*), his classical prose. TCM holds that the heart plays a dominant role in the vital activity of the whole body, so it is called "monarch". These unpleasant things can easily hurt one's mind.

------ 健康小提示 ----------------------------- **Health-preserving Tips**

劳逸结合有益健康,同时,不要因为小事而心烦气躁。

Striking a proper balance between work and rest is good for health. At the same time, don't get upset or irritable because of trivial matters.

3　身怕不动,脑怕不用。

Both the body and the brain need to be used.

俗语说:"身怕不动,脑怕不用。"一个人不劳动、不运动是很可怕的。至于大脑,它是人体的总指挥官,更是要充分使用起来。脑子是越用越灵的,如果一段时间不动脑思考,人的反应就会变得迟钝,甚至会得阿尔茨海默病。

As the saying goes, both the body and the brain need to be used. It's terrible that one doesn't work or exercise. As for the brain, the commander in chief of the human body should be fully used. The more one uses his/her brain, the smarter he/she will be. If one doesn't use his/her brain for a period of time, his/her reaction will become dull, and one may even get Alzheimer's disease.

------ 健康小提示 -- **Health-preserving Tips**

医学研究证明人类在生活中,勤奋工作,积极创造新鲜事物,可以刺激脑细胞再生,并恢复大脑活力,所以,动脑是延缓人体衰老的有效方法。但大脑又不宜过度使用,要注意合理用脑。

Medical research has proved that human beings work hard and actively create new things in life, which can stimulate brain cell regeneration and restore brain vitality. Therefore, brain movement is an effective way to delay human ageing. On the other hand, the brain should be used properly rather than overused.

4 神大用则竭,形大劳则敝,形神离则死。

When *shen* (spirit) is overused, one will go to exhaustion, when physique is overused, one will feel tired, and when both of them are overused, one will die.

精神过度使用就会走向衰竭,身体过度劳累就会感觉疲惫,精神与身体都疲累不堪时,人就会死亡。心情愉快,身体健康,人才能长寿。

When *shen* (spirit) is overused, one will go to exhaustion, when physique is overused, one will feel tired, and when both of them are overused, one will die. Good mood and healthy body can make one live longer.

------ 健康小提示 -- **Health-preserving Tips**

日常生活中不论遇到多么复杂的事情,都要保持乐观的处世态度,顺应事物自身的发展规律去解决问题。

No matter how complex things one encounters in his/her daily life, he/she should maintain an optimistic attitude, and solve the problems according to the development laws of things.

5　动则不衰，乐则长寿。

Exercise and happiness make a young man.

"动"和"乐"是保持健康的两个关键，老年人的生活乐趣比年轻人少，很容易心情抑郁，不想运动，身体便会处于亚健康状态。心理压力过大会造成精神疲劳，身体免疫力下降。

"Exercise" and "happiness" are the two keys to health preservation. The elderly have less fun in life than the young. They are prone to feel depressed and do less exercise, and their bodies will be in sub-health condition. Excessive psychological pressure will cause mental fatigue and reduce the body's immunity.

----- 健康小提示 -------------------------------- **Health-preserving Tips**

运动不宜过量，最好在稍微感到疲劳时停止。

One should not exercise too much. It's best to stop when one feels a little tired.

6　养生之道，常欲小劳。

Proper amount of work is beneficial to health.

中国唐代著名的医药学家孙思邈在《备急千金要方》中提出"养生之道，常欲小劳"。生活中运动过量会导致排汗过多而损伤阳气。

Sun Simiao, a famous Chinese pharmacist in the Tang Dynasty, put forward "Proper amount of work is beneficial to health" in *Bei Ji Qian Jin Yao Fang* (*Golden Prescriptions for Emergency Use*). Excessive exercise can cause excessive sweating and damage *yang qi* of the body.

----- 健康小提示 -------------------------------- **Health-preserving Tips**

劳动可以把毒素通过汗水从体内排泄出来，促进人体新陈代谢。要注意，过度劳作会损耗人的精力，对人体健康有害。

Labor can excrete toxins from human body through sweat and promote human body's metabolism. It should be noted that overwork will deplete

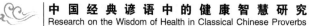
one's energy and is harmful to human health.

7　天天练长跑，年老变年少。

Long-distance running every day makes one young.

俗语说："天天练长跑，年老变年少。"专家认为，在所有运动中，跑步最影响人的寿命。跑步可以快速消除人的不良情绪。经常跑步的人，身体和心理素质都很高，寿命也更长。

As the saying goes, "Long-distance running every day makes one young." Experts believe that running affects one's lifespan the most among all sports. One who runs regularly will live longer. Running can eliminate one's bad emotions quickly. One who runs regularly has high physical and mental qualities and lives longer.

------ 健康小提示 ------------------------------ **Health-preserving Tips**

长跑可以对心脏循环系统产生有益的影响，并能提高能量基础代谢和免疫力。要注意，跑步时要采用正确的姿势和呼气方法。

Long-distance running has a beneficial effect on the heart circulatory system. It can also improve the basic energy metabolism and immunity. The correct posture and exhalation method should be adopted when running.

8　运动好比灵芝草，何必苦把仙方找。

Physical exercise is the best medicine.

本谚语强调应经常进行适度运动。不同于一般药物对某种疾病起治疗作用，亦不同于一般保健食品只对某一方面营养素的不足进行补充和强化，运动是在整体上调节人体功能平衡，调动机体内部活力，调节人体的新陈代谢功能，提高免疫力，促使全部器官的功能正常化，如同传说中有神奇作用的灵芝草。

This proverb emphasizes that moderate exercise should be carried out frequently. Unlike general medicines that can treat certain diseases or general health foods that only supplement and strengthen a certain aspect of nutrient deficiency, exercise regulates human functions in general, adjusts the body's internal vitality, regulates the body's metabolic function, improves the immunity, and promotes the normalization of all internal organs. It is like the magical *lingzhi* (Ganoderma) in the legend.

------- 健康小提示 ------------------------------ **Health-preserving Tips**

灵芝是一味应用范围非常广泛的中药,所治病种涉及呼吸、消化、神经和循环系统。灵芝可以增强人体免疫力。

Lingzhi is a traditional Chinese medicine with a very wide range of applications. It treats diseases involving respiratory, digestive, nervous, and circulatory systems, and can strengthen human immunity.

9　动以健身,静以养心。

Activities help to keep fit and inertia helps to nourish the heart.

健身的关键是动静结合。运动能增强我们的心肺功能,改善血液循环系统。人摒除一切杂念,才能进入天人合一的境界之中,怡养心神。

The key to fitness is the combination of proper exercise and rest. Doing exercise can enhance one's cardiorespiratory function and improve the blood circulation system. Only when one get rid of all distracting thoughts can he/she enter the realm of the unity of man and nature and nourish his/her mind.

------- 健康小提示 ------------------------------ **Health-preserving Tips**

对老年人来说,静比动更重要。此外,老年人运动,不可骤起或骤停。老年人的阴、阳之气都须慎重保护。

For the elderly, rest is more important than exercise. In addition, the elderly should not start or stop suddenly when exercising. Both *yin qi* and *yang qi* of the elderly should be carefully protected.

10 养花就怕不浇水,运动就怕不久长。

If one grows flowers, he/she should water them on time; if one does exercise, he/she should stick to it for a long time.

运动养生的持续性十分重要。大家都知道运动有益健康,尝试通过运动来养生健身的人也不计其数,但并不是每个人都能从中受益。"三天打鱼,两天晒网"是无法达到养生效果的。

The continuity of health preserving with exercise is very important. Everyone knows that exercise is good for health, and there are countless people who try to keep fit through exercise, but not everyone can benefit from it. Exercising by fits and starts can't achieve the purpose of health preserving.

----- 健康小提示 ----------------------------- **Health-preserving Tips**

可以找一个志同道合且意志坚定的朋友一起运动,互相监督,提高运动的热情,避免半途而废。

One can find a like-minded and determined friend to exercise together and supervise each other, which can improve the enthusiasm of sports and avoid giving up halfway.

第二节 动静结合
Section Two Association of Activity and Inertia

1 早起做早操,一天精神好。

Get up early and do morning exercises, and one will be energetic all day.

人睡眠过后体力会得到恢复,但机体仍然处于一定的抑制状态。要想尽快摆脱精神不振的状态,起床后做早操是一种很好的办法。做早操,可以加快身体各部分机能的恢复速度,呼吸新鲜空气有助于振作精神,从而为一天的劳动或学习提供充分精力。

One's physical strength will recover after sleep, but the body is still in a certain state of inhibition. In order to recover from the state of low spirits as soon as possible, it is a good way to do morning exercises after getting up. Doing morning exercises can speed up the recovery of the functions of all parts of the body. Breathing fresh air helps one to cheer up, so as to prepare enough energy for a day's work or study.

----- 健康小提示 -------------------------------- **Health-preserving Tips**

早晨的运动量不宜过大,以免身体过分疲乏,影响一天的劳动和学习。

One should not exercise too much in the morning so as to avoid excessive fatigue and adverse effects on work and study during the day.

2　有静有动,无病无痛。

We can keep in good health with activity and inertia.

动静结合是运动养生中一个非常重要的观点。许多专家都认为只有将动养生和静养生结合起来才能帮助身体达到最佳状态。

Association of activity and inertia is highly recommended in exercise regimen. Many experts believe that only combining the methods of dynamic health-preserving and static health-preserving can people keep in good health.

----- 健康小提示 -------------------------------- **Health-preserving Tips**

在传统养生的运动中,太极拳讲究动静结合,以"慢""静"为主,也有"静"转"动"的出拳姿势。在武术中,动静结合被称为练功的最高境界。

In the traditional health keeping exercise, *taijiquan* stresses the association of activity and inertia, with "slowness" and "stillness" as the main body, and also has the boxing posture of "stillness" to "movement". In martial arts, the combination of movement and stillness is called the highest level of exercise.

3 饭后百步走,活到九十九。

A walk after meals promises a long life.

饭后散步能够促进消化,有助于控制血糖。在进食完以后,应该起身进行散步等简易活动。这里所说的"饭后百步"并不提倡饭后急行,而是缓行,不宜缓行者也应该多摆动手足。

Walking after meals can promote digestion and help control blood sugar. One should stand up for a walk and other simple activities after a meal. The activities mentioned don't mean rushing after a meal, but walking slowly. Those who are not suitable for walking can also shake their hands and feet.

------ 健康小提示 ------------------------------ **Health-preserving Tips**

要注意,体质较差特别是患有胃下垂等病的人,不适合饭后散步,最好在饭后平卧10分钟。因为饭后胃内食物充盈,此时如果进行直立性活动,会加重胃的负担。患有冠心病、心绞痛、贫血、低血压的人饭后应该先按摩腹部,休息半小时后再进行散步活动。

It should be noted that people with poor physique, especially those with gastroptosis, are not suitable for walking after meals. It is better for them to prostrate for 10 minutes after meals because the stomach is full of food after a meal. At this time, if people do upright activities, the burden on the stomach will be increased. People suffering from coronary heart disease, angina pectoris, anemia and hypotension should massage their abdomen after meals and take a walk after half an hour's rest.

4 久坐伤肉,久卧伤气,久立伤骨。

Sitting for a long time impairs the muscle; sleeping for a long time impairs *qi*; standing for a long time impairs the bone.

《黄帝内经》有说:"久坐伤肉,久卧伤气,久立伤骨。"这句谚语点明了长期保持坐、卧、立等静止状态的弊端,从而强调了运动在气血保养方面的益处。适当的运动和劳作会让人精神百倍。

In *Huang Di Nei Jing* (*Huangdi's Canon of Medicine*), it is said that sitting for a long time impairs the muscle; sleeping for a long time impairs *qi*; standing for a long time impairs the bone. This proverb points out the disadvantages of maintaining a static state such as sitting, lying, and standing for a long time, thereby emphasizing the benefits of exercise in nourishing *qi* and blood. Appropriate exercise and work will make people more energetic.

------ 健康小提示 ------------------------------ **Health-preserving Tips**

每坐半个小时,应该起身运动一次,做一些类似伸懒腰、扩胸、抬头、走动的小动作,有益健康。

One should stand up and exercise after sitting for half an hour. Doing movements like stretching, expanding the chest, raising the head, and walking are good for one's health.

5 劳逸相宜。

All work and no play makes Johnny a dull boy.

劳逸结合是最常见的养生做法;作息不规律对身体有较大的损害。

Striking a proper balance between work and rest is the most common health regimen. Irregular work and rest have great damage to the body.

------ 健康小提示 ------------------------------ **Health-preserving Tips**

人们最好在 23 点前睡觉,一旦超过这个时间,人体气血循环便会受到影响,更不利于五脏的养生,对健康有很大危害。

People had better go to bed before 23 o'clock, or their blood circulation will be influenced. Staying up late is not conducive to the health preserving of the five *zang* viscera and is very harmful to health.

6 行走疾如风,血脉上下通。

A brisk walk keeps the blood vessels unobstructed.

快步走是一种十分简便的运动养生方法,可以贯通全身血脉,使人体气血畅通。快步走时全身骨骼所受到的冲击力比较小,与站立或散步时区别不大。另外,快步走还可以预防中老年人易得的骨质疏松症。

Brisk walking is a simple exercise regimen that can make blood vessels unobstructed. The impact on the bones of the whole body is relatively small when walking briskly, which is not much different from that when standing or walking. In addition, brisk walking can also prevent osteoporosis that the old are prone to incur.

------ 健康小提示 ------------------------------ **Health-preserving Tips**

快步走前一定要做一会儿热身动作,避免造成运动损伤。注意要选择平坦开阔的场地,防止被障碍物绊倒。

One should warm up for a while before brisk walking to avoid athletic injuries, and he/she had better choose a flat site to prevent tripping over obstacles.

7 大步走,小步跑,一天万步比较好。

Striding and jogging about ten thousand steps would be better for health.

走路是一种增强体质和免疫力的理想运动方法。步行和跑步有益心脏健康,不仅可以减肥瘦身,还能让人体充满能量,这些都可以起到延长寿命、提升生活质量的作用。此外,步行还可以缓解我们的心理压力。

Walking is an ideal exercise method to enhance our physical fitness and immunity. Walking and running are good for heart's health. It can not only help us lose weight, but also increase our vitality, which can prolong life and improve the quality of life. In addition, walking can also relieve one's psychological pressure.

------ 健康小提示 ---------------------------------- **Health-preserving Tips**

跑步时穿合适的跑鞋,可以缓冲脚底的压力。长距离走路前一定要做一些准备活动,如轻轻压压肌肉和韧带,做一些下蹲运动等,让自己的心脏和肌肉进入到运动状态。

Wearing suitable running shoes when running can cushion the pressure on the soles of your feet. Before a long walk, one must do some preparatory activities, such as gently pressing the muscles and ligaments and doing some squatting exercises to get his/her heart and muscles into the state of exercise.

8　常运动,骨头硬。

Regular exercise helps to harden the bones.

骨头硬就是骨密度增加,不管是哪一种锻炼,只要能持之以恒,对提高骨密度都是有效的。增加骨密度的最佳运动是负重和跳跃。

To make the bone hard is to increase the bone mineral density. Any kind of exercise is effective to improve the bone mineral density as long as one keeps doing. The best exercise to increase BMD is weight-bearing and jumping.

------ 健康小提示 ---------------------------------- **Health-preserving Tips**

要想使骨头变硬,提高骨骼里的含钙量,一定要保证饮食中的钙含量。多晒太阳,吃点维生素 D 可以促进钙的吸收。

If one wants to harden his/her bones and increase the calcium content in the bones, he/she must ensure the calcium content in the diet, get more exposure to the sun and eat vitamin D to promote calcium absorption.

9　好饭莫饱。

Don't eat too much no matter how delicious the food is.

美味的饭菜,不能吃得太饱,否则会伤胃。吃得太饱的话,不仅会引起肥胖,还会造成胃下垂,胃里的食物残渣还可能引起便秘、口臭等一些消化系统疾病。

Don't overeat even though the food is delicious, or it will hurt the stomach. If one eats too much, it will not only cause obesity, but also cause stomach ptosis. Food residues in the stomach may also cause constipation, foul breath and other digestive diseases.

------ 健康小提示 -------------------------- **Health-preserving Tips**

不要暴饮暴食。吃饭时要专注于食物,不要边吃饭边看书或者看电视,否则容易导致肠胃供血不足,不利于消化。

Don't overeat. When one eats, he/she should focus on food. Don't read books or watch TV while eating. Otherwise, it's easy to make the blood supply of intestines and stomach insufficient, which is not conducive to digestion.

10 没事常走路,不用进药铺。
Walking often keeps the doctor away.

散步是一种协调性运动,坚持散步可以使周身的肌肉收缩,促进血液和淋巴系统循环,加速代谢,增强免疫力。人们早晨起床后应该到庭院里走一走,适当活动筋骨。

Walking is a kind of coordinated exercise. Persisting in walking can contract muscles of the whole body, promote the circulation of blood and lymphatic system, accelerate metabolism and enhance immunity. When one gets up in the morning, he/she should take a walk in the courtyard and exercise properly.

------ 健康小提示 -------------------------- **Health-preserving Tips**

当心情特别低落时,出去走会儿路,可以很有效地调节情绪。

When one is particularly depressed, go out for a while and relax, which can effectively regulate his/her mood.

11　要使腿不废,走路往后退。
Walking backwards makes one's legs more flexible.

倒行运动有助于我们维持腿脚的正常生理功能,避免老年人容易出现的退行性改变,可预防颈椎病、腰椎病、肩周炎等,有效改善腰肌劳损,放松处于紧张状态的肌肉与骨骼。在倒着走路的过程中,需要抬头挺胸,这样有利于提高脊柱的承受能力,有效防止佝偻或驼背。

Walking backwards helps us maintain the normal physiological functions of one's legs and feet, avoids the degenerative changes that are prone to the elderly, prevents cervical spondylosis, lumbar spondylosis and frozen shoulder, effectively improves lumbar muscle strain, and relaxes muscles and bones under tension. In the process of walking backwards, one needs to raise his/her head and chest, which helps to improve the bearing capacity of the spine and effectively prevents rickets or hunched back.

----- 健康小提示 ---------------------------- Health-preserving Tips

倒着行走时一定要找一片没有危险障碍物的场地。走路过程中集中注意力可以有效预防阿尔茨海默病。要注意,长时间倒着走路会使膝盖的负荷量增大。

When walking backwards, be sure to find a field free of dangerous obstacles. Concentrating attention during walking can effectively prevent Alzheimer's disease. It should be noted that walking backwards for a long time will increase the load on the knees.

12　若要身体健,天天来锻炼。
Exercising every day makes one healthy.

锻炼身体可以促进身体的血液循环以及新陈代谢,使身体处于一个良好的状态,避免一些代谢性疾病和免疫性疾病的发生。此外,锻炼身体还能够开发身体的潜能,比如心脏和肺的功能,有助于人体适应一些较为恶劣的环境。

Exercising can promote the blood circulation and metabolism of the body, keep the body healthy, avoid some metabolic diseases and immune diseases. In addition, exercising can also develop the body's potential, such as the function of the heart and the lung, and help the body adapt to the harsher environments.

----- 健康小提示 ---------------------------------- **Health-preserving Tips**

不要在晚上九点以后锻炼身体，否则会影响睡眠质量。

Don't exercise after 9 p. m. , or the sleeping quality will decline.

13 卫生是妙药，锻炼是金丹。

Hygiene and exercise are both important to keep healthy.

卫生与健康息息相关，不讲卫生的人容易生病。锻炼可以促进脂类的代谢，有利于血管保持弹性，预防高血压、糖尿病，使身体处于一个良好的状态，可以更高效地工作。

Hygiene and health are closely related. People who pay no attention to hygiene tend to get sick. Exercising can promote the metabolism of lipids, help maintain the elasticity of vessels, avoid high blood pressure and diabetes, and make one in a good condition to work more efficiently.

----- 健康小提示 ---------------------------------- **Health-preserving Tips**

厨房里准备两个菜板，不要用同一个菜板切蔬菜和生肉。

It's very important to prepare two chopping boards in the kitchen. Don't cut vegetables and raw meat on the same board.

14 跑步虽有益，并非都适宜。

Running is good for health, but it does not fit everyone.

跑步锻炼是人们最常采用的一种身体锻炼方式。它不需要特殊的环境，又是一种全身运动，能使全身的肌肉有节律地收缩和松弛，使肌肉纤维增多，蛋白质含量增高。室外跑步能增加血液中氧气的携带量，改善心脏功能，使皮肤、肌肉变得更加有弹性、有力量，延缓衰老。但跑步并非适合所有的人。罗圈腿、X型腿、膝关节损伤、体重过大的人群不适合跑步，建议选择其他运动方式。

Running exercise is the most commonly used way of physical exercise. It does not need a special environment. What's more, it is a holistic exercise, which can make the muscles of the body contract and relax rhythmically, increase the muscle fiber and protein content. Outdoor running can increase the amount of oxygen carried in the blood, improve heart function, make skin and muscles stronger, and delay aging. But running is not suitable for to everyone. People with cirded legs, X-shaped legs, knee joint injuries and excessive weight had better not run. It is recommended for them to choose other sports.

----- **健康小提示** ----------------------- **Health-preserving Tips**

跑步的运动量过大,心脏病患者和严重高血压患者不适宜跑步。

People with heart disease and severe hypertension should not run because it takes too much energy.

15　水不动生毒,人不动生病。

Stagnant water will produce toxins while inactive people will get sick.

本谚语强调运动对人体健康的作用。流动中的水含氧量高,可以促进污染物的分解。不流动的水含氧量少,反过来促进水中厌氧性生物的增长,产生许多有害物质。人在运动时呼吸加快,排汗增多,有利于体内代谢废物或有毒物质的排泄。

This proverb emphasizes the effect of exercise on human health. The flowing water has high oxygen content, which can promote the decomposition of pollutants. Stagnant water contains less oxygen, which in turn promotes the growth of anaerobic organisms in water and produces many harmful substances. Exercise makes people breathe faster and sweat more, which is conducive to the excretion of metabolic wastes or toxic substances in the body.

----- **健康小提示** ----------------------- **Health-preserving Tips**

美国运动学者泰勒指出,轻快散步或做其他的温和运动,可以使身心产生一种全面性的转变。

Taylor, an American sports scholar, pointed out that brisk walking or other mild exercise can make a comprehensive change to the body and mind.

16 铁不炼不成钢，人不运动不健康。
Iron needs to be calcined repeatedly to become stronger steel; people need exercise to be healthy.

本谚语用铁要经过反复煅烧才能变成更为坚韧的钢来形容运动要持之以恒。进行适度的有规律的运动，可以给健康带来极大的好处。人不运动，血流运行会减慢，肺活量会减弱，不利于体内代谢废物的排泄。

In this proverb, "Iron needs to be calcined repeatedly to become stronger steel" is used to compare "exercising should be persevered". Moderate and regular exercise is good for health. If people don't exercise, the blood flow will slow down and the vital capacity will weaken, which is not conducive to the excretion of metabolic waste in the body.

------ 健康小提示 ------------------------------ **Health-preserving Tips**

坚持不懈地进行有氧运动，可使呼吸、循环、消化、神经、内分泌、运动等各系统器官得到自然的刺激，促进青少年生长发育，使中年人保持旺盛的精力，使老年人衰老的速度减慢。总之，要想身体健康，离不开适当的运动。

Persistent aerobic exercise can stimulate the respiratory, circulatory, digestive, nervous, endocrine, sports and other organs naturally, promote the growth and development of teenagers, keep the middle-aged energetic, and slow down the aging speed of the elderly. In a word, one can't be healthy without proper exercise.

17 蹦蹦跳跳筋骨壮，萎萎缩缩百病生。
Jumping makes one strong and recoiling makes one ill.

运动有益于人体健康，而萎靡不振只会对身体造成损伤。做运动伸展身体可以缓解疲劳，加速体内代谢循环，使体内废物迅速排出体外。

Exercise is good for one's health, and lethargy will only do harm to one's body. Taking exercise and stretching can relieve fatigue, accelerate the metabolic cycle in the body, and make the waste be discharged from the body quickly.

------ **健康小提示** ------------------------------- **Health-preserving Tips**

早上起来活动活动筋骨,对人体大有益处。每天待在室内不运动,会引起多种慢性病。

Doing morning exercise is good for one's health. Staying indoors every day without exercise will cause a variety of chronic diseases.

18　松腰练腿好,九十也不老。

Relax the waist and exercise the legs, and one won't get old even at 90 years old.

正确的姿势可以提高运动的质量。松腰指腰椎及其韧带,腰两侧肌肉等都放松,逐步改变腰部的自然弯曲状态;练腿常用的方法是压腿。应遵循由低到高、由易到难的原则,切忌蛮压暴拉,造成不必要的肌肉和软组织损伤。

Correct posture can improve the quality of exercise. Loosing waist refers to the lumbar spine and its ligaments, and muscles on both sides of the waist are relaxed, changing the natural bending state of the waist gradually. The common method for leg training is to press the legs. One must follow the principle of from low to high, from easy to difficult, and avoid excessive pressure and violent pulling, which may cause unnecessary muscle and soft tissue damage.

------ **健康小提示** ------------------------------- **Health-preserving Tips**

酒后不宜健身。酒精会使人兴奋,所以有人酒后会去健身消耗多余的精力。然而酒后健身会加大肝脏的压力,同时会损伤大脑。

It is not suitable to keep fit after drinking. Alcohol can make one excited, so some people will go to gym after drinking to consume extra energy. However, doing exercise after drinking will increase the pressure on the liver and cause brain damage.

19 年轻勤锻炼，老来身体健。

One will be healthy when he/she is old if he/she does exercise regularly when he/she is young.

年轻时多锻炼身体，到年老时身体就会健康。如果年轻时只顾每天拼命工作，而从不锻炼身体，年老时可能会得慢性病和疑难病。年轻人必须要从现在开始锻炼身体，才能健康地退休，安享晚年。

One will be healthy when he/she is old if he/she does exercise regularly when he/she is young. If one only works hard every day when he/she is young and never exercises, he/she may get chronic diseases and difficult diseases when he/she is old. Young people must exercise from now on to retire healthily and enjoy their old age.

----- 健康小提示 ------------------------------- Health-preserving Tips

很多年轻人觉得自己年轻有活力，就从不去锻炼身体，再加上经常作息不规律，进行高强度的工作，久而久之各种健康问题就会产生，而花费大量的时间、金钱和精力在医院是得不偿失的。

Many young people think that they are young and energetic, so they never take exercise. In addition, they often work and rest irregularly and do high-intensity work, which will lead to various health problems over time. It's not worth spending a lot of time, money and energy in the hospital.

20 运动有益，过量有害。

Exercise is good for health, but excessive exercise will have a counterproductive effect.

运动有益于身体和精神健康。它能减少许多疾病，如心脏病、癌症、糖尿病的发生率；有利于维持健康的体重。但是过度运动不但消耗糖类和脂肪，还消耗蛋白质，反而会有害于人体的健康。老年人的体力和身体机能与年轻人相比有所衰退，更是要适量运动。

Exercise is good for physical and mental health. It can reduce the incidence of many diseases, such as heart disease, cancer and diabetes, and help maintain a healthy figure. However, excessive exercise not only consumes sugar and fat, but also consumes protein, which will be harmful to human health. The physical strength and physical functions of the elderly are declining compared with those of the young, and it is more necessary for them to exercise appropriately.

----- 健康小提示 ------------------------------ **Health-preserving Tips**

大量运动会使人体产生的一种作用类似吗啡的物质增加。这种物质若释放到血液中,会使人感到兴奋,可抑制各种不适与疼痛。一旦停止运动,便会使人产生沮丧、易激动、焦虑不安的感觉。

A large amount of exercise will increase a substance similar to morphine produced by the human body. If this substance is released into the blood, it will make people feel excited and can inhibit all kinds of discomfort and pain. Once stop exercising, one will feel depressed, irritable and anxious.

21 练出一身汗,小病不用看。

People who often sweat through exercise don't have to go to the hospital for a minor illness.

俗话说:"练出一身汗,小病不用看。"现在也流行一句话"请人吃饭不如请人流汗"。对于工作压力大的上班族来说,运动出汗对身体很重要。人们身体排泄废物的途径除了大小便外就是出汗。现代人缺乏运动,出汗非常少,体内的毒素容易沉积下来,破坏身体正常状态,时间长了就会生病。

As the saying goes, "People who often sweat through exercise don't have to go to the hospital for a minor illness." There is also a popular saying now, "Inviting someone to eat is not as good as inviting someone to sweat." For office workers with high pressure, sweating due to exercise is good for us. People excrete waste from their bodies mainly through urination and sweating. Modern people lack exercise and seldom sweat. The toxins in the body are easily deposited, destroying the normal state of the body, and making people sick over time.

------ 健康小提示 ------------------------------ **Health-preserving Tips**

现代社会环境污染问题严重,人们更需要多运动来出汗排毒,但是不能过度出汗,否则会损伤人体的阳气。

The environment today is often heavily polluted, and people need more exercise to sweat and detoxify. But people had better not sweat too much, otherwise it will damage *yang qi* in the body.

22 心灵手巧,动指健脑。

The more fingers exercise, the more flexible the brain is.

从中医经络来说,手指的经络系统连接着大脑,所以动动手指,就会有刺激大脑神经,使大脑细胞活跃的作用。老年人经常锻炼手指,还可以预防阿尔茨海默病的发生。

From the perspective of meridians in TCM, the meridian system of fingers is connected to the brain, so exercising fingers can stimulate the brain nerves and activate the brain cells. Elderly people can exercise their fingers regularly to prevent Alzheimer's disease.

------ 健康小提示 ------------------------------ **Health-preserving Tips**

要培养手指的灵活性,可以用指尖从事一些比较精细的活动,例如拼装乐高,每天练习一会儿,就可以起到健脑的作用。

To cultivate the flexibility of fingers, one can use his/her fingertips to do some relatively precise activities, such as assembling LEGO. It only takes a short time every day to build our brain and body.

23 常练筋长三分,不练肉厚一寸。

One should exercise regularly, which will increase the length of tendon, otherwise it will increase the thickness of meat.

现代人大多过于重视肌肉的锻炼,而忽视了"筋"的锻炼。中医学认为,筋不单是指经络,还包括现代医学中的韧带、骨骼肌等部位。筋附着在骨头上,具有收缩肌肉、联络关节、固定骨骼等作用。

Most modern people pay much attention to muscle training and neglect the training of tendons. According to TCM, tendons not only refer to meridians, but also include ligaments and skeletal muscles in modern medicine. Tendons are attached to bones, which can contract muscles, connect joints and fix bones.

----- **健康小提示** ------------------------------ **Health-preserving Tips**

武术和瑜伽等运动都有助于筋的锻炼。拉筋后饮用一杯温开水,有利于人体的气血运行。

Martial art, yoga and other sports are conducive to the training of tendons. Drinking a cup of warm water after stretching is beneficial to the operation of *qi* and blood in one's body.

24　白天多动,夜间少梦。

The more one exercises during the day, the less he/she dreams at night.

白天多运动,有助于晚上睡眠。如果我们在白天从事较多的体力和脑力劳动,身体感到疲乏,晚上躺在床上很快便能睡着,并且起床后精力充沛。相反,白天无所事事的人,晚上就会很难入睡。

Exercise during the day helps to improve the quality of sleep at night. If one does more physical and mental work during the day, he/she will feel tired and fall asleep quickly when he/she lies in bed at night. What's more, he/she will be energetic on the next day. On the contrary, those who are idle during the day will have difficulty in sleeping at night.

----- **健康小提示** ------------------------------ **Health-preserving Tips**

中医认为,人最好在晚上九点至十一点入睡。

TCM believes that it is the best time for us to go to bed between 9 o'clock and 11 o'clock in the evening.

第三节　特色养生
Section Three　Characteristic Health Preserving

1　小便不通阴陵泉。

Massaging Point *Yinlingquan* helps to urinate smoothly.

人们在夏天很容易受暑湿之邪的伤害而感冒或拉肚子。针对暑湿之邪的特点,人们首先要保持身体的气血正常,因为气血不足或过盛的时候,人体抵抗力就会降低。每天坚持按揉阴陵泉有助于人们在夏天脾胃消化功能正常。

People are prone to get cold or diarrhea in summer due to summer-damp pathogen. According to the characteristics of summer-damp pathogen, people should first keep their *qi* and blood normal. Because when the *qi* and blood are insufficient or excessive, people's immunity will be reduced. Pressing and kneading Point *Yinlingquan* (SP 9) every day can ensure the normal digestive function of spleen and stomach in summer.

------ 健康小提示 ------------------------------ **Health-preserving Tips**

阴陵泉是足太阴脾经的一个穴位,其具体位置在小腿的内侧,胫骨内侧髁下方的凹陷处。

Point *Yinlingquan* (SP 9) is a acupuncture point in the spleen meridian of foot *taiyin* (SP), which is located in the inner side of the leg and the depression under the medial condyle of tibia.

2　常按足三里,胜吃老母鸡。

Massaging Point *Zusanli* will let one benefit more even than drinking old hen soup.

中医里讲,鸡肉能补肾益精、补益脾胃、补血养阴,可用于治疗阳痿、遗精、少精、食欲不振、面色萎黄、产后体虚、头晕、闭经等。老母鸡的补益作用更高,对于病久体虚的人颇为适宜。后来,人们在不断与疾病作斗争的过程中,发现经常按摩足三里有益健康,故有"常按足三里,胜吃老母鸡"一说。

TCM believes that eating chicken can tonify kidney and essence, spleen and stomach, blood and *yin qi*, and can be used to treat impotence, spermatorrhea, oligospermia, loss of appetite, sallow complexion, postpartum body deficiency, dizziness, amenorrhea, etc. The tonic effect of old hen soup is higher, which is quite suitable for people with chronic disease and weakness of body. Later, in the process of constantly fighting against diseases, people found that massaging Point *Zusanli* (ST 36) has the similar effect with eating chicken, Therefore, there is a saying that "Massaging Point *Zusanli* will let one benefit more even than drinking old hen soup."

----- 健康小提示 ---------------------------- **Health-preserving Tips**

用手掌覆于膝盖上,五指朝下,中指指尖向外一指的位置就是足三里穴。

Cover the knee with the five fingers facing down, and the tip of the middle finger is pointing outwards at Point *Zusanli* (ST 36).

3 锻炼按摩练气功,健康长寿活百岁。
People who exercise, massage and practise *qigong* can live a long and healthy life to 100 years old.

按摩可以疏通经络,使气血周流,保持机体的阴阳平衡。经常练习气功,不仅能够帮助人们改善血液循环,有效地提高人体的免疫力,还可以缓解器官的衰老,对保证身体健康有重要作用。

Massage can dredge the meridians, make blood flow around, and maintain the balance of *yin* and *yang* in the body. Regular practice of *qigong* can not only help people improve blood circulation and the immunity, but also reduce the aging process of the organs, which plays an important role in ensuring physical health.

----- 健康小提示 ---------------------------- **Health-preserving Tips**

早晨、中午最好在饭前练气功,使胃脏被气场作用之后再行进食。

It is best to practice *qigong* before meals in the morning and at noon, so that the stomach can be affected by the *qi* field before eating.

4 饭后千步走，常以手旋腹。

Walking after meals and rubbing your stomach often are good for health.

此谚语所讲的是饭后养生的方法：饭后散步与旋腹，有益于食物消化，其中饭后散步是广为人知的日常养生之道，而旋腹则并不十分普及，但事实上，以手旋腹不仅同样简便易行，而且对促进食物消化更有奇效。

This proverb describes the method of health preservation after a meal: walking after a meal and massaging abdomen are good for digestion. Walking after a meal is a well-known health regimen in people's daily lives. Massaging abdomen is not very popular, but in fact, it is not only easy and convenient, but also effective in promoting digestion.

----- 健康小提示 ----------------------------------- **Health-preserving Tips**

饭后半小时走路能促进食物消化，但不可急步快走。

Walking half an hour after a meal can promote digestion, but people should not walk quickly.

5 老人多摇扇，筋骨更舒展。

The elderly can stretch their muscles and bones by shaking fans.

在很多人的心目中，一位老人坐在椅子上不快不慢地摇着手中的扇子是长寿老人的一个典型形象。此谚语中提到了扇子除了散热的日常用途之外，另一种特殊的用途是舒展筋骨。摇扇子不仅仅是日常生活中的一个小习惯，更是一项简便的养生动作。

Many people think that an old man sitting in a chair and shaking the fan in his hand is a typical image of a long-lived old man. This proverb states that fans can not only be used to dissipate heat, but also help people stretch their body. Shaking the fan is not only a small habit in daily life, but also a simple exercise for health-preserving.

摇扇子时最好左右手替换着摇,能同时刺激左右脑,有利于心脑血管健康。

Shaking the fan with two hands in turn can stimulate the left and right brains at the same time, which is conducive to cardiovascular and cerebrovascular health.

6　常伸懒腰乃古训,消疲养血又养心。
Stretching can eliminate fatigue, nourish blood and heart.

伸懒腰人人都会,这个简单的动作却具有保养气血、消除疲劳的神奇作用,正如谚语中所说:"消疲养血又养心。"中医认为,伸懒腰是人体一种自我调节的方式,伸懒腰时双手上举,体内的器官因此都得以舒张,具有调节胃气、舒理三焦的作用。

Stretching is a simple action that everyone can do. It has magical effect of maintaining *qi* and blood and eliminating fatigue. Just as the saying goes, "Stretching can eliminate fatigue, nourish blood and heart." TCM believes that stretching is a way of self-regulation of the human body. When one lifts his/her hands, all the organs in the body can be relaxed, which has the function of regulating stomach *qi* and relaxing triple energizer.

长时间坐立、不锻炼,会导致小腿部位肌肉萎缩,而在伸懒腰过程中,全身肌肉都会在一定时间内保持比较紧张的状态,此时小腿部位肌肉会由于长期紧张而出现痉挛。

Sitting for a long time without exercising will cause muscle atrophy in the calf. During the stretching process, the muscles of the whole body will remain relatively tense for a certain period of time. At this time, the muscles of the calf will have spasm due to long-term tension.

7 摩热脚心能健步。

Rubbing the soles of the feet can increase walking speed.

搓脚心能使脚部毛细血管扩张,加快血液循环,供给脚部更多的能量和氧气,使腿脚的新陈代谢能力更加旺盛。脚心上有许多神经直接连接大脑,搓脚心可以刺激脚心神经,使大脑感到轻松,不管是体力劳动者还是脑力劳动者,每晚睡前搓搓脚心都能消除疲劳。

Rubbing the soles of the feet can expand the capillaries of the feet, speed up blood circulation, supply more energy and oxygen to the feet, and make the metabolism of the legs and feet more vigorous. There are many nerves in the soles of the feet that are directly connected to the brain. Rubbing the soles of the feet can stimulate the nerves and make the brain relaxed. Rubbing the soles of the feet every night can eliminate fatigue for most people, whether they are manual workers or mental workers.

------ 健康小提示 ----------------------------- **Health-preserving Tips**

最好饭后一小时以后再按摩脚心,同一部位连续按摩时长不要超过 5 分钟。

Don't massage the soles of the feet within one hour after a meal, and don't massage the same part for more than 5 minutes.

8 要想能多活,按摩涌泉穴。

Massaging Point *Yongquan* can extend one's life.

涌泉穴在脚心上,它是足少阴肾经的起点,按摩此穴,具有滋阴补肾的作用。老年人常按摩这一穴位,还能缓解腿脚麻木、行动无力等。

There is a Point *Yongquan*（KI 1）on the center of the foot, which is the starting point of the kidney meridian of foot *Shaoyin*（KI）and is important for health-preserving. Massaging at this point can nourish *yin* and kidney. Frequent massaging of the soles of the feet can also help the elderly relieve the numbness and weakness of their legs and feet.

------ **健康小提示** ----------------------------- **Health-preserving Tips**

按摩涌泉穴有助于扩张血管、促进血液循环、加快毒素排出、降低血液黏稠度。

Massaging the Point *Yongquan*（KI 1）can help one dilate blood vessels, promote blood circulation, speed up the discharge of toxins, and reduce blood viscosity.

9　要想全身少得病，勤揉耳朵与聆听。

Frequent ear rubbing and listening help one reduce the chance of getting sick.

俗话说："要想全身少得病，勤揉耳朵与聆听。"中医学认为耳朵与脏腑、经络关系密切。现代医学也认为，经常按摩耳朵，有助于强身健体、防病治病、延年益寿。

As the saying goes, "Frequent ear rubbing and listening help one reduce the chance of getting sick." TCM believes that ears are closely related to *zang-fu* organs and meridians. Modern medicine also believes that regular ear massage can help to strengthen the body, prevent and treat diseases and prolong life.

------ **健康小提示** ----------------------------- **Health-preserving Tips**

平时工作压力大的人，可以在上班途中揉一揉、拉一拉自己的耳朵。每天只需花几分钟，不仅可减轻身体的不适症状，还能使人精神振奋。

People with high work pressure can use their time on the way to work to rub and pull their ears. It only takes a few minutes every day, which can not only reduce the physical discomfort, but also boost the spirit.

10　跑步打拳舞剑，健康要靠锻炼。

Running, boxing and sword dancing are good for health.

到户外进行跑步、打拳、舞剑、做健身操、爬山或去公园散步等活动，可以迅速消除身体疲劳,舒展肢体的活动还能促进脾胃功能恢复。

Outdoor activities such as running, boxing, sword dancing, doing aerobics, mountain climbing or going for a walk in the park can quickly eliminate physical fatigue, stretch limbs and promote the recovery of spleen and stomach function.

----- 健康小提示 ----------------------------- **Health-preserving Tips**

过度疲惫时不宜进行剧烈运动,室内办公人员最好利用休息时间去室外走走。

People should not take strenuous exercise when they are too tired. Indoor office workers had better take a walk outside during their break time.

11　打拳击剑,寿增一半。
Boxing and fencing can prolong life.

打拳可以提高自身的反应能力,促进身体健康以及宣泄情绪。击剑会使人的姿态更优雅。击剑需要不断地观察,不断地思考,在进入交锋距离内,在有限的时间里,要迅速做出反应,从而形成一种全新的思维模式,有助于身心健康。

Practicing boxing can help one improve reaction capability, promote health and vent emotions. Fencing will make one more elegant. When one is fencing, he/she needs to constantly observe, constantly think, and quickly respond within the distance and in the limited time, so as to form a new mode of thinking, which is conducive to physical and mental health.

----- 健康小提示 ----------------------------- **Health-preserving Tips**

击剑打拳前要规范穿戴护具,否则很容易受伤。

One should wear protective gear rightly before fencing and boxing, otherwise it is easy for him/her to get injured.

12　食毕摩腹,百病能除。
Massaging the abdomen after meals can cure the diseases.

饭后用手轻轻按摩腹部,能加快腹腔内血液循环,加强胃部功能,对老年人的健康大有裨益。作为一种良性刺激,食后摩腹有益于神经、体液内分泌功能的调节,且能活血通络、疏通经脉,对肠胃和心脑血管系统疾病有独特的防治作用。

Massaging the abdomen gently after meals can promote the blood circulation in the abdominal cavity and strengthen the function of the stomach, which is of great benefit to the health of the aged. As a kind of benign stimulation, massaging the abdomen after meals is beneficial to the regulation of neuroendocrine and humoral endocrine function. It can also activate blood circulation, dredge main meridians. It has a unique preventive and therapeutic effect on gastrointestinal and cardiovascular diseases.

----- 健康小提示 ----------------------------- **Health-preserving Tips**

过度饥饿或暴食后都不宜按摩腹部。

One should not massage the abdomen after excessive hunger or overeating.

13 按摩劳宫,精神轻松。

Massaging Point *Laogong* makes one more energetic.

经常刺激劳宫穴,可疏通心包经,具有镇静安神、健脑益智和强壮心脏的功效。有口臭症状时,多按这个穴位,能起到缓解的作用。

Stimulating Point *Laogong* (PC 8) frequently can dredge the pericardial meridian. It has the effects of calming the nerves, invigorating the brain and strengthening the heart. It can also relieve the bad breath.

----- 健康小提示 ----------------------------- **Health-preserving Tips**

中暑或者晕车时,按揉劳宫穴有明显的缓解效果。

When one has heatstroke or motion sickness, rubbing Point *Laogong* can relieve the symptoms effectively.

14   脚膝经年痛不休,内外踝边用意求。

Massaging Point *Kunlun* can relieve the lasting pain of leg and foot.

昆仑穴在五行中属于火,对应的是心,膀胱经经别入于心,心藏神,故按摩此穴有助于治疗神志病。而且按摩昆仑穴能够疏通经络、消肿止痛,对腿足红肿、脚踝疼痛治疗效果良好。

Point *Kunlun* (BL 60) is attributed to the fire in the five elements, corresponding to the heart, the bladder meridian enters the heart, and heart stores the spirit, so massaging this point can help treat mental illness. In addition, massaging Point *Kunlun* (BL 60) can dredge the meridian, reduce swelling and relieve pain and has a good effect on the treatment of leg and foot swelling and ankle pain.

------ 健康小提示 ------------------------------- **Health-preserving Tips**

按摩昆仑穴有缓解头痛的作用,对于保护视力也有一定的好处。

Massaging Point *Kunlun* (BL 60) can relieve headache and protect the eyesight.

15   腰背委中求。

Massaging Point *Weizhong* can relieve low back pain.

委中穴是中医针灸经络中的四大总穴之一。按摩委中穴有舒筋通络、散淤活血、清热解毒的功效。

Point *Weizhong* (BL 40) is one of the four command points in the acupuncture meridian of TCM. Massaging Point *Weizhong* (BL 40) has the effect of relaxing tendons and dredging meridian, activating blood to resolve stasis, clearing heat and relieving toxin.

------ 健康小提示 ------------------------------- **Health-preserving Tips**

正确地按摩承山穴和昆仑穴也能很好地解除腰背的酸痛。

Massaging Point *Chengshan* (BL 57) and Point *Kunlun* (BL 60) can also relieve low back pain.

16 头项寻列缺。

Massaging Point *Lieque* can cure headache.

所有头部的疾病如头疼、头晕等,都可以用按摩列缺穴来治疗。由于列缺属于肺经上的要穴,所以按摩它还能治疗与肺相关的疾病,如咳嗽、气喘、咽喉肿痛等。

All head diseases, such as headache and dizziness can be treated with massaging Point *Lieque* (LU 7). Because Point *Lieque* (LU 7) belongs to the important points on the lung meridian, it can also treat diseases related to lung, such as cough, asthma, sore throat, etc.

------ **健康小提示** --------------------------------- **Health-preserving Tips**

按摩列缺穴直到有酸胀感时最有效。

It is the most effective to massage Point *Lieque* (LU 7) until one has a sense of soreness.

第四章　养生谚语四季篇

Chapter Four　Health-preserving Proverbs About Four Seasons

第一节　春季养生

Section One　Health Preserving in Spring

1　缓解春困小妙招,吃葱杀菌抗疲劳。

Eating green onions helps to kill bacteria and resist fatigue.

　　一到春天很多人都提不起精神,加上春季细菌过度滋生,疾病也容易发生,春季多吃点葱,有杀菌抗疲劳的功效。葱含有的挥发油和辣素可以祛除饭菜中的腥、膻等异味,产生特殊香气,并有较强的杀菌作用。挥发性辣素通过汗腺、呼吸道、泌尿系统从体内排出时会轻微刺激相关腺体,起到发汗、祛痰、利尿的作用,在治疗感冒方面有一定功效。

　　Many people are not energetic in spring. In addition, there is excessive breeding of bacteria in spring and diseases are also prone to occur. Eating more green onions in spring can kill bacteria and relieve fatigue. The volatile oil and capsaicin contained in green onions can remove fishy, mutton and other peculiar smells in meals, produce a special aroma, and have a strong bactericidal effect. When volatile capsaicin is discharged from the body through the sweat glands, respiratory tract, and urinary system, it will slightly stimulate related glands, play the role of sweating, dispelling phlegm, and diuretic, and have certain effects on the treatment of colds.

葱虽有益健康,但是过量食用可能会损伤视力。此外。葱对汗腺具有较强的刺激作用,有腋臭的人在夏季尽量少吃。

Although green onions are good for health, excessive consumption may damage eyesight. In addition, green onions have a strong stimulating effect on sweat glands, so people with underarm odor should eat as little as possible in summer.

2　春天放风筝,祛病又健身。
Flying kites in spring can cure diseases and keep fit.

春天,晴空碧净,鸟语花香,正是放飞风筝的好时节。此时去放风筝,不仅给生活增添了许多乐趣,而且对人的身体健康是非常有益处的。中医认为,放风筝者沐浴和煦的阳光和温暖的春风,有疏泄内热、增强体质之益。

In spring, the sky is clear and blue, and the birds and flowers are fragrant. It is a good time to fly kites. Flying a kite at this time not only adds a lot of fun to life, but also is very beneficial to people's health. TCM believes that the warm sunshine and spring breeze can relieve kite-flyers' internal heat and enhance their physical fitness.

放风筝应选择空旷处,避免障碍物,切勿在有高压线电塔、有电线杆架设施处放。放风筝时要留意气候变化,如有台风、雷击现象,应马上停止施放并远离空旷处。

When flying a kite, one should choose an open area to avoid obstacles. People should not fly kites in places where there are high-voltage line towers or telegraph poles. One should pay attention to climate changes before flying. If there are typhoons or lightning strikes, one should stop flying at once and stay away from the open area.

3 春天喝碗河蚌汤,不生痱子不长疮。

Drink mussel soup in spring can prevent rash and sore.

清明前的河蚌最干净,肉质最肥厚,这个时节吃河蚌有清热解毒、滋阴凉血、养肝明目之功效,适合阴虚内热之人,也适宜糖尿病、尿路感染、甲状腺机能亢进、高血压、湿疹、癌症等患者食用,其还有预防起痱子的作用。

The mussels in the period before the Qingming Festival are the cleanest and most nutritious. Eating mussels at this time can clear heat and relieve toxin, nourish *yin* and cool blood, nourish the liver and improve eyesight. It is suitable for people with *yin* deficiency and internal heat, as well as for patients with diabetes, urinary tract infection, hyperthyroidism, hypertension, eczema, cancer, etc. It can also prevent prickly heat.

----- 健康小提示 ------------------------------ **Health-preserving Tips**

蚌肉性寒,因此脾胃虚弱的人不能食用。要学会挑选活的河蚌来进行烹饪,因为死的河蚌的肉易分解产生腐败物,细菌会繁衍得特别快,若食用了死的河蚌,极有可能会招致食物中毒,引起肠胃类疾病。

Mussel meat is cold in nature, so people with asthenia of spleen and stomach shouldn't eat it. People should learn to choose live mussels for cooking, because the meat of dead mussels is easy to decompose and produce spoilage, and bacteria will multiply fastly. If people eat dead mussels, they are very likely to incur food poisoning and gastrointestinal diseases.

4 春捂秋冻,不生杂病。

If one dresses thicker in spring and thinner in autumn, he/she won't get sick easily.

"春捂秋冻,不生杂病"是自古以来就流传着的养生保健谚语。春季气候变化反复无常,人们应该注意保暖;秋季阳始退而阴渐长,要适当少穿些衣服;这样做可以增强人体对气候变化的适应能力,有助于机体的健康。

"If one dresses thicker in spring and thinner in autumn, he/she won't get sick easily" is a popular health-preserving proverb since ancient times. People should keep warm because of the changeable climate in spring. *Yang* begins to recede and *yin* grows in autumn. People should wear less clothes in this season. This can enhance people's ability to adapt to climate change and contribute to people's health.

------ 健康小提示 ----------------------------------- **Health-preserving Tips**

老年人和儿童免疫力比较低,不适合秋冻。另外,有支气管病、哮喘病、冠心病的人不宜秋冻。

The immunity of the elderly and children is relatively low, so they should not dress thinner. In addition, people with bronchial disease, asthma and coronary heart disease should not dress thinner in autumn.

5　春季进补汤,祛寒数鸡汤。

It is suitable to drink tonic soup in spring, and chicken soup has the best effect on wiping off the chill.

春季是一个滋补身体的好时节,鸡汤为春季进补第一汤。鸡汤有温中益气、补虚填精、活血脉、强筋骨的功效。鸡汤蛋白质含量高,且易被人体消化吸收,能提高免疫力,防治感冒,有助于减少咳嗽次数、减轻鼻塞和咽喉疼痛感。

Spring is a good time to nourish the body, and chicken soup can be the first tonic soup in spring. Chicken soup has the effects of warming and replenishing *qi*, tonifying weakness and essence, activating blood vessels, and strengthening muscles and bones. Chicken soup is rich in protein and is easy to be digested and absorbed by the human body. It can also improve immunity, prevent and treat colds, help reduce the severity of cough, and relieve nasal congestion and sore throat.

------ 健康小提示 ---------------------------- **Health-preserving Tips**

高血压、高血脂、胆囊炎、急慢性肾功能不全和胃溃疡患者不适合喝鸡汤。

Patients with hypertension, hyperlipidemia, cholecystitis, acute and chronic renal insufficiency, and gastric ulcer shouldn't drink chicken soup.

6　三月三,荠菜当灵丹。

Shepherd's purse at March 3 is like a kind of precious medicine.

中医认为荠菜可用于治疗痢疾、水肿、淋病、吐血、便血、血崩、月经过多等。现代医学研究也证实,荠菜中含有乙酰胆碱、丰富的维生素 C 和胡萝卜素等,具有很高的营养价值,是不可多得的药食同源之物。荠菜含有大量的粗纤维,食用后可增强大肠蠕动,促进排泄,有助于防止高血压、冠心病、肥胖症、糖尿病、肠癌及痔疮。

TCM believes that shepherd's purse can be used to treat dysentery, edema, gonorrhea, vomiting blood, blood in the stool, bleeding, and menorrhagia. Modern medical research has also confirmed that shepherd's purse contains acetylcholine, rich vitamin C and carotene, etc. It has high nutritional value and is a rare medicinal and food homolog. Shepherd's purse contains a lot of crude fiber. It can enhance the peristalsis of the large intestine, promote excretion, and help prevent high blood pressure, coronary heart disease, obesity, diabetes, bowel cancer and hemorrhoids.

----- 健康小提示 ----------------------------- **Health-preserving Tips**

荠菜根的药用价值很高,食用时不应摘除。荠菜不宜久烧久煮,加热时间过长会破坏其营养成分,也会使其颜色变黄。荠菜可宽肠通便,便溏者慎食。体质虚寒者不能食用荠菜。

Shepherd's purse root has a high medicinal value and should not be removed when eating. Shepherd's purse should not be heated for a long time, otherwise its nutrients will be destroyed and its color will turn yellow. Shepherd's purse can relax the bowel, and those who have loose stools should be cautious in eating it. People with weak constitution can not eat shepherd's purse.

7　春游去踏青，春暖防过敏。

People should prevent allergies when going out in spring.

　　春天百花盛开，是外出踏青、享受明媚阳光的大好时机。但是，每当春暖花开之际，花粉在空气中飘散时，很容易被人吸进呼吸道内，有过敏体质者吸入这些花粉后，就会产生过敏反应。

　　The flowers are in full bloom in spring, which is a great time for people to go out and enjoy the bright sunshine. However, when the flowers bloom, the pollen is dispersed in the air. It is easy to be inhaled into the respiratory tract. People with allergies will have allergic reactions after inhaling the pollen.

------ **健康小提示** ---------------------------- **Health-preserving Tips**

　　人们可以去医院做血清特异性过敏源检测，以帮助判断是否属过敏体质。过敏体质的人应多吃水果蔬菜，如富含维生素 A 的胡萝卜等，不宜吃易致皮肤过敏的虾蟹类食品。

　　People can go to the hospital for serum-specific allergen testing to help determine whether they are allergic. People with allergies should eat more fruit and vegetables, such as vitamin A-rich carrots. It is not advisable for them to eat shrimps and crabs that can easily cause skin allergies.

8　春来哪有不食葱。

Eat more green onions in spring is good for health.

　　春天的葱是一年中营养最丰富，也是最嫩、最香、最好吃的时候。此时生长出来的葱，由于气候和土壤的关系，不仅仅是香料，还是特殊的补品。它可以帮助人们恢复身体机能，补给热量。贫血、低血压和怕冷的人，更应该多吃。春季气候变化无常，感冒发生率高，此时多吃些葱，可以缓解病情，并可预防春季呼吸道感染。

　　In spring, green onions are the most nutritious, tender, fragrant, and delicious of the year. Green onions grown at this time are not only spices, but also special tonics due to the climate and soil. They can help people restore their body functions and replenish calories. People with anemia, low blood pressure, and fear of cold, should eat more green onions. The climate is changeable in spring, and the incidence of colds is high. At this time, eating more green onions can alleviate the disease and prevent respiratory tract infection in spring.

葱不适宜和蜂蜜一起食用,因为蜂蜜中含有的一些酶会和葱发生反应,从而产生一些对我们身体有害的成分,严重的话还可能导致腹泻或者胃痛。

Green onions shouldn't be eaten with honey, because honey contains some enzymes that can react with green onions to produce some harmful ingredients. In severe cases, it may cause diarrhea or stomach pains.

9 春不食肝,夏不食心。

One should not eat the liver in spring, and should not eat the heart in summer.

春季肝气旺,此时吃肝会使肝气更旺,容易出现脾胃虚弱症状。动物肝脏富含维生素 A,大量摄入会导致头晕、头疼、过敏及腹泻等中毒症状。夏至开始宜进行饮食调养,炎夏时心火当令,所以有"夏不食心"的说法。

In spring, the liver *qi* is vigorous. Eating liver at this time will lead to exuberance of liver *qi*, and people are prone to have asthenia of spleen and stomach. The animal liver is rich in vitamin A, which can lead to dizziness, headache, allergy and diarrhea. At the beginning of the Summer Solstice, one had better take good care of himself/herself by eating. In the hot summer, the heart fire is in season, so there's a saying that "don't eat the heart in summer".

动物肝脏胆固醇含量很高,沉积在血管壁上的胆固醇,容易引发血管粥样硬化,故老年人应少吃。

Cholesterol content in animal liver is very high. Cholesterol deposited in the wall of blood vessels is easy to cause atherosclerosis, so the elderly should eat less.

10　春天孩儿脸，一天变三变。

The climate is changeable in spring.

这条谚语说的是春天气候的多变性。虽然春季逐步回暖，但早晚温差较大，不时还会出现倒春寒。若气温突然下降，人体将难以适应，病菌则会攻击身体，容易引发各种呼吸道疾病及春季传染病。

This proverb points out the variability of spring climate by means of metaphor. Although it is gradually warming up in spring, the temperature difference between morning and evening is large, and sometimes there will be late spring cold. If the temperature drops suddenly, it will be difficult for the human body to adapt, and the bacteria will attack the body and easily cause various respiratory diseases and spring infectious diseases.

------ *健康小提示* ----------------------------- **Health-preserving Tips**

春天气候多变化，要根据天气变化，适时增减衣服，否则出汗以后更加容易着凉感冒。春季人体的各个器官、组织、细胞的新陈代谢开始旺盛起来，正是锻炼的好时机。

The climate in spring is changeable. One should change clothes in time according to the weather change. Otherwise, he/she will be more likely to catch cold after sweating. The metabolism of various organs, tissues and cells of the human body begins to be more vigorous in spring, which is a good time for exercise.

11　春天冻人不冻水。

People will feel cold in spring, but the water won't freeze.

春天，太阳光的热先照射到地面上，被地面吸收，地面上的温度升高后，热量再传给空气，所以空气中的热量是间接从太阳光中得到的。靠近地面的空气温度更高，冰雪便开始融化。冰雪在融化的过程中要吸收热量，降低了地面温度的升高速度。冰雪融化以后，空气中的湿度增大，带走人体表面的热量，人们便会感觉到冷。

In the spring, sunlight first shines on the ground, and the heat is absorbed by the ground. After the temperature on the ground rises, the heat is transferred to the air, so the heat in the air is obtained indirectly from the sun. The air near the ground becomes hotter, then the ice and snow begin to melt. Ice and snow absorb heat in the process of melting, reducing the rate of increase in ground temperature. After the snow melts, the humidity in the air increases, taking away the heat from the surface of the human body, and people will feel cold.

----- 健康小提示 ----------------------------- Health-preserving Tips

春天不要着急脱掉棉衣,以免着凉。对于老年人来说,室温最好保持在15℃以上。

One should not take off his/her cotton clothes in a hurry in spring to avoid getting cold. For the elderly, they had better keep the room temperature above 15℃.

12　春风吹日暖,春燥早日防。

The wind in spring is warm, but don't forget to prevent dryness in spring as soon as possible.

春天风邪侵袭人体,人体的防护功能减弱,较难保持体内新陈代谢的平衡和稳定,易扰动人体肝、胆、胃肠,蓄积内热,出现春燥。春燥形成的另一个原因是在漫长的冬季,人们往往穿着厚厚的棉衣,喜欢吃热气腾腾的饭菜来抵御严寒的侵袭。一些上了年纪的人还经常喝点酒,吃一些温热的滋补品。这些在冬季看来是必要的,但会使人体内积蓄较多的郁热,需要早点预防。

In spring, wind pathogen invades the human body, and the protective function of the human body is weakened, which makes it difficult to maintain the balance and stability of the body's metabolism. The pathogen tends to disturb the liver, gallbladder, and gastrointestinal tract, accumulate internal heat, and cause dryness in spring. Another reason for the formation of dryness in spring is that people usually wear thick cotton clothes, eat steaming meals to resist the invasion of the cold in winter. Some elderly people even often drink wine and eat warm tonics.

These habits seem to be necessary in winter, but they can also accumulate more stagnant heat in the body and need to be prevented in advance.

------ 健康小提示 ------------------------------------- **Health-preserving Tips**

预防春燥可以多吃新鲜的水果蔬菜,同时注意生活规律,保持心情愉快,提高身体免疫力。

To prevent spring dryness, one can eat more fresh fruit and vegetables, live a regular life and keep a happy mood to improve body immunity.

13　春季养生当食补,辛甘温食为上选。
One can nourish the body by eating bland food in spring.

由于气候变化无常,老年人在春季容易生病。根据中医病理学,春补原则以清淡为宜。适量吃些甜食还可以调动脾胃活力。多吃新鲜蔬菜,可以补充维生素。

The elderly are easy to get sick in spring because of the changeable climate. According to the pathology of TCM, the principle of tonic in spring should be bland. Eating some sweet food in moderation can also strengthen the function of spleen and stomach. Fresh vegetables can supplement the vitamins that people need.

------ 健康小提示 ------------------------------------- **Health-preserving Tips**

用红枣、黄芪煮水,每天饮用可提高免疫力,预防疾病来袭。

Putting red dates and *huangqi* (milkvetch root) together to make a soup and drinking it every day can improve immunity and prevent diseases in spring.

14　百草回芽,百病易发。
The grass sprouts and people get sick easily in spring.

春天是"百草回芽,百病易发"的季节。清明节气以前气温变化较大,这段时间人体最容易受到风邪的侵袭,因此很多疾病容易在春季发作,特别是心血管疾病和流感。

The grass sprouts and people get sick easily in spring. The temperature changes greatly before the Qingming solar term. The human body is most susceptible to the invasion of wind pathogen during this period. Therefore, many diseases, especially cardiovascular disease and influenza, tend to occur in spring.

----- **健康小提示** ----------------------------------- **Health-preserving Tips**

开窗通风是最简单的居室消毒方法,但是日出前与傍晚是两个污染高峰,要避开这两个时间段开窗。常戴口罩不仅可以防沙尘,还可以预防流感和过敏。

Opening windows for ventilation is the easiest way to disinfect the room, but there are two peaks of pollution before sunrise and evening, so people should not open windows during these two periods. Wearing a mask often can not only keep out sand and dust, but also prevent flu and allergies.

15　春困秋乏夏打盹,睡不醒的冬三月。

One is prone to sleep in spring and cold winter, feel tired in autumn, and drowse in hot summer.

春天,天气逐渐变暖,人们会感到困倦、疲乏、昏昏欲睡;夏天,受气温和人体自身因素的影响,身体各器官的功能在白天会处于一种困倦状态;秋天,天气逐渐变冷,人容易精神不振,想要睡觉;冬天,生命活动处于极度降低的状态,以应对外界寒冷的环境。

People will feel sleepy, tired and drowsy in spring when the climate is getting warmer; in summer, affected by temperature and human body's own factors, the function of body organs is in a sleepy state in the daytime; in autumn, the weather gradually becomes cold, people tend to be depressed and want to sleep; in winter, life activities are extremely reduced to cope with the cold environment.

----- **健康小提示** ----------------------------------- **Health-preserving Tips**

冬天温度较低,血液循环速度减慢,人们容易疲倦,每天晚上最好能休息八个小时,睡眠时间也不宜过长,否则同样会导致白天没有精神。

The temperature is low in winter. Blood circulation slows down, and people get tired easily. It is best to rest for eight hours every day, and the sleep time should not be too long, otherwise it will also cause drowsiness during the daytime.

16　四时百病，胃气为本。

Stomach *qi* plays an important role in maintaining human health.

这句话强调了"胃气"在生命活动中的重要性，只有胃气强才能抵抗各种疾病。胃气不足，则进入人体的食物不能被充分消化吸收，反而在肠胃中堆积，从而出现消化不良、食欲不振等症状，各个器官也得不到充足的养分，免疫力便会降低。相反，若是胃气过盛，就会出现恶心、打嗝、胃液逆流等肠胃症状。在这种情况下，食物也不能被完全转化为营养素，不仅造成营养浪费，还会造成肠胃疾病。

This sentence emphasizes the importance of "stomach *qi*" in life activities. Only strong stomach *qi* can resist various diseases. If the stomach *qi* is insufficient, the food entering the human body cannot be fully digested and absorbed. Instead, it accumulates in the intestines and stomach, resulting in indigestion, loss of appetite and other diseases. The organs cannot get sufficient nutrients, and the immunity will be reduced. On the contrary, if the stomach *qi* is excessive, one will incur nausea, hiccups, reflux of gastric juice and other gastrointestinal symptoms. In this case, food can not be completely converted into nutrients, which not only results in a waste of nutrition, but also causes gastrointestinal diseases.

----- 健康小提示 ----------------------------- **Health-preserving Tips**

中医认为，舌苔是由胃气所生，因此观察舌苔可判断胃气是否充足。正常情况下舌上均有白色薄苔。

TCM believes that the tongue coating is produced by stomach *qi*, so observing the tongue coating can determine whether the stomach *qi* is sufficient. Normally there is a thin coating on the surface of the tongue.

第二节　夏季养生
Section Two　Health Preserving in Summer

1　六月六，晒衣服，减少疾病添幸福。

Sunning clothes on June 6 can reduce the incidence of diseases and increase happiness.

衣服要在天气好的时候多拿出来翻晒，太阳光中的紫外线可起到消毒杀菌的作用。用木棒或者其他物体拍打衣物可以使衣物上的粉尘落地，同时拍打可以使衣物变得蓬松，衣物的内部间隙增大，更利于空气在衣物间流通。

Clothes should be taken out when the weather is good. The ultraviolet light in the sunlight can play the role of disinfection and sterilization. Beating clothes with sticks or other objects can make the dust fall to the ground. At the same time, beating can make the clothes fluffy and increase the internal gap of the clothes, which is more conducive to the air circulation between the clothes.

----- 健康小提示 ---------------------------- **Health-preserving Tips**

衣物晒得过度的话，会损伤衣服的颜色和质地。
Sunning too long may damage clothes' color and quality.

2　夏季多吃蒜，消毒又保健。

Eating more garlic in summer is helpful for disinfection and health-preserving.

夏天天气炎热，细菌容易滋生繁殖，吃点大蒜，可以避免得肠炎、痢疾等胃肠道疾病。许多研究证明，大蒜具有很强的抗菌作用，对于肠道内大肠杆菌、痢疾杆菌的抑制作用尤为显著，所以，大蒜在民间有"天然抗生素"之称。

It's hot in summer, and bacteria are easy to breed. Eating garlic can help people avoid enteritis, dysentery and other gastrointestinal diseases. Many studies have proved that garlic has a strong antibacterial effect, especially for the inhibition of escherichia coli and dysentery bacilli. Therefore, garlic is known as "natural antibiotic" in the folk.

------ **健康小提示** ------------------------------- **Health-preserving Tips**

长期大量吃蒜对眼睛有害。

Eating garlic in large quantities for a long time is harmful to eyes.

3　夏练三伏降酷暑，冬练三九傲霜寒。

One should insist on physical exercise no matter how cold or hot the weather is.

不管天气多冷或多热，人们都应坚持体育锻炼，这样才能使身体更好地适应四季气温。在炎热的夏季，越不活动，人体适应外界环境的能力就越差。适当锻炼，能使皮下毛细血管扩张，加快腺体开放速度，提高身体散热能力，增强人体体温调节能力。

No matter how cold or hot the weather is, people should insist on physical exercise, so that the body can better obtain the ability of "adapting to the temperature of four seasons". In the hot summer, the more inactive the body is, the worse one can adapt to the external environment. Proper exercise in a hot environment can make subcutaneous capillaries dilate, speed up the opening of body glands, improve the body's ability of heat dissipation and enhance the ability to regulate temperature.

------ **健康小提示** ------------------------------- **Health-preserving Tips**

运动不能过量，冬天要防寒保暖，夏天要防止中暑。

Excessive exercise is not advisable. One should keep warm in winter and prevent heatstroke in summer while exercising.

4 夏不睡石,秋不睡板,春不露脐,冬不蒙头。

One should not sleep on rocks in summer, or sleep on boards in autumn, or show the navel when sleeping in spring, or cover the head when sleeping in winter.

夏天躺在石头上睡觉虽然凉爽但容易感冒,裸着背睡在石头上还可能会损伤背部。秋天不睡木板,是因为木板太硬,不利于人体的血液循环,于养生无益。初春相对来说还是有点冷的,睡觉时没有盖好被子,并且把肚脐露出来的话很有可能会着凉并且感冒。冬天把头蒙在被子里睡觉,严重影响吸入空气的质量,第二天还会感觉头脑昏沉,影响工作效率。

Although it's cool to sleep on a stone in summer, it's easy to catch a cold. Sleeping on a stone with naked back may cause back injury. The reason why one should not sleep on a board in autumn is that the board is too hard, which is not conducive to the blood circulation of the human body and is not benefit to health preservation. It is relatively cold in early spring. If one doesn't cover the body properly and expose the navel when sleeping, he/she is likely to catch a cold. Sleeping with the head covered in the quilt in winter will seriously affect the quality of the inhaled air, and he/she will feel dizzy the next day, which will reduce work efficiency.

------ 健康小提示 ------------------------------ **Health-preserving Tips**

坚持早睡早起,适量室外运动能预防感冒。

Going to bed early, getting up early and going out for proper exercise can prevent colds.

5 立夏日,吃补食。

People should eat nourishing food at the beginning of summer.

立夏吃蛋能使心气精神不受亏损,强健身体。吃竹笋是希望双腿像春笋那样健壮有力。豌豆形如眼睛,吃豌豆是为了祈盼眼睛清澈明亮。在立夏吃这些食物,往往寄托着人们祈福保平安的愿望。

At the beginning of summer, eating eggs can protect the mind and spirit and strengthen the body. Eating bamboo shoots means that people want their legs to be as powerful as spring bamboo shoots. Peas are shaped like eyes. Eating Peas is to pray for clear and bright eyes. At the beginning of summer, eating these foods often reposes people's desire to pray for peace and happiness.

---- 健康小提示 ------------------------------ **Health-preserving Tips**

立夏日应该吃咸鸭蛋,其中红心咸蛋更是久负盛名,它美味可口,清香四溢,富有营养,老少皆宜,咸鸭蛋的钙含量比鲜蛋高很多。

One should eat salted duck eggs at the beginning of summer. Red heart salted eggs are even more well-known. They are delicious, fragrant, nutritious, and suitable for all ages. The calcium content of salted duck eggs is much higher than that of fresh eggs.

6 贪凉失盖,不病才怪。

Sleeping without a quilt will cause illness.

睡觉时为了凉爽而不盖被子,很容易着凉生病。当我们睡觉时,身体器官都处于休眠期。人体脏器对温度非常敏感,即便在非常热的时候,也会因受凉发生腹痛、腹泻。胸背还有很多重要穴位,受凉后容易发生胃肠道、呼吸道和心血管疾病。长此以往,身体血管会发生萎缩,导致免疫机能下降。

One is prone to catch a cold if he/she doesn't cover the guilt while sleeping. When one is sleeping, his/her organs are dormant. Human organs are very sensitive to temperature. Even when it is very hot, abdominal pain and diarrhea will occur due to cold. There are also many important acupoints on the chest and back, which are prone to gastrointestinal, respiratory and cardiovascular diseases after catching a cold. Over time, the blood vessels will atrophy, leading to a decline in immune function.

---- 健康小提示 ------------------------------ **Health-preserving Tips**

夏天晚上睡觉时,最好不要一直开空调和风扇,也不要对着窗户睡觉。盖一

个薄毛毯,这样可以避免着凉。

In summer, one had better not keep the air conditioner or electric fan on while sleeping, and should not sleep in front of the open window. He/She had better cover a thin blanket to avoid catching a cold.

7　汗水没干,冷水莫沾。

One should not touch cold water until the sweat has evaporated.

人体在出汗时,皮肤下的毛细血管和皮肤上的毛孔都处于扩张状态,以利于汗液的排除和机体热量的发散。此时如果直接接触凉水,就会导致机体血管受到极大的刺激,皮肤毛孔也会随之快速收缩,不利于健康。

When the human body perspires, the capillaries under the skin and the pores on the skin are in a state of expansion, which is conducive to the elimination of sweat and the divergence of body heat. At this time, if one directly contacts with cold water, body's blood vessels will be greatly stimulated, and the skin pores will contract rapidly, which is harmful to health.

------ 健康小提示 ----------------------------- **Health-preserving Tips**

运动后可以用毛巾先擦去身上的汗液,待汗水完全干后,再用温水洗澡,达到清洁降温的目的。可以喝一杯淡盐水,在补水的同时也补充盐分。

After doing exercise, one can wipe the sweat off the body with a towel, wait until the sweat is completely evaporated, and then take a bath with warm water to achieve the purpose of cleaning and cooling. One can drink a cup of light salt water to replenish the salt of body.

8　立夏开始喝姜茶,三伏就喝黄芪粥。

One can drink ginger tea when summer begins, and *huangqi* (milkvetch root) porridge on dog days to build the body.

人们在夏天喜欢吃冷的食物,并且待在阴凉的环境中,这非常容易损伤脾胃,引发腹痛、腹泻等疾病。姜茶有防治感冒、健脾暖胃、活血化淤等功效,产妇、脾胃虚的人都可以喝。中气不足的人，最适宜用黄芪进补。

People like to drink cold drinks in summer and stay in a cool environment. The spleen and stomach are therefore easily damaged, causing abdominal pain, diarrhea and other diseases. Ginger tea has the effects of preventing and treating cold, strengthening spleen and warming stomach, and promoting blood circulation and removing stasis. Parturients and people with asthenia of spleen and stomach should drink more ginger tea. *Huangqi* (milkvetch root) is the most suitable tonic for people with insufficient *qi*.

----- **健康小提示** ---------------------------- **Health-preserving Tips**

做黄芪粥时，要注意黄芪本身是不能吃下去的。

It is necessary to understand that *huangqi* (milkvetch root) itself cannot be eaten if one wants to make *huangqi* porridge.

9　天时虽热，不可食凉；瓜果虽美，不可多尝。

Don't eat cold food no matter how hot it is; don't eat too much melon and fruit no matter how delicious it is.

夏天很多人得肠胃炎，是吃过多冰凉的东西造成的。中医认为夏天人的阳气往外走，如果吃凉的东西太多，肠胃便会发僵，蠕动能力减弱，人的吸收功能也会受损。平时脾胃虚弱的人更少吃瓜果，而且，瓜果一定要新鲜。

Many people get gastroenteritis in summer, which is caused by eating too much cold food. TCM believes that people's *yang qi* goes out in summer. If they eat too much cold food, their stomach will become stiff, their peristaltic ability will be weakened, and their absorption function will be impaired. People with asthenia of spleen and stomach should eat melon and fruit sparingly. Moreover, the melon and fruit must be fresh.

----- **健康小提示** ---------------------------- **Health-preserving Tips**

胃溃疡、胃炎、消化不良患者不宜吃冷饮。儿童消化功能尚未发育完善，多吃生冷食物，尤其是糖分高的冰激凌、饮料等，易损伤脾胃的运化功能。

Patients with gastric ulcer, gastritis, and dyspepsia should not eat cold drinks. Since children's digestive function is not yet well-developed, eating more raw and cold foods, especially ice creams and drinks with high sugar content, can easily damage their spleen and stomach's function of transportation and transformation.

10　暑天吃西瓜，药剂不用抓。

Eat watermelon in summer, and keep away from medicine.

大热天吃西瓜，不但可饱人口福，而且还有很好的养生保健作用。西瓜甘甜多汁，所含果汁是所有瓜果中最为丰富的，既可解渴利尿，又可去暑散热，素有"瓜果之王"的美称。

Eating watermelon in hot weather can not only satisfy people's appetite, but also be beneficial to the health. Watermelon is sweet and juicy. Its juice is the most abundant among all melon and fruit. It can not only relieve thirst and diuresis, but also dissipate summer heat. It is known as "the king of melon and fruit".

----- 健康小提示 ---------------------------------- **Health-preserving Tips**

脾胃虚寒者不宜多吃西瓜，否则易引起腹胀、腹泻和食欲下降；糖尿病患者和口腔溃疡者过量食用西瓜会加重病情。

People with asthenia of spleen and stomach should not eat too many watermelons, otherwise they may incur abdominal distension, diarrhea and loss of appetite. The condition of the patients with diabetes and oral ulcer may worsen if they eat too many watermelons.

11　夏天一碗绿豆汤，解毒去暑赛仙方。

Drinking mung bean soup in summer helps to detoxify and drive away summer heat.

绿豆不仅是一种食物，更是一剂良好的解毒去暑中药。中医认为，绿豆味甘、性寒，有利水消肿、清暑止渴等功效，常用于治疗暑热、丹毒以及小便不利。

Mung bean is not only a kind of food, but also an effective detoxification and anti-heat Chinese medicine. TCM believes that mung beans are sweet in taste and cold in nature, and are beneficial to water detumescence, heat clearing and thirst quenching. It is often used in expelling summer heat, erysipelas and urinary problems.

----- 健康小提示 ----------------------------------- **Health-preserving Tips**

绿豆性凉,脾胃虚弱的人不宜多吃。服药特别是服温补药时不要吃绿豆食品,以免降低药效。

The mung bean is cool in nature. People with asthenia of spleen and stomach had better not eat too many mung beans. When taking medicine, especially warming and tonifying medicine, people should not eat mung bean food so as not to reduce the efficacy.

12 六月韭,驴不瞅。

Leeks in June are not palatable.

韭菜性温,可以补益肾气,旺盛精力。春天人体肝气偏盛,木克脾土,因此会影响脾胃的运化功能,食用韭菜刚好可以增强脾胃之气。但是到了夏天,特别是到了6月份,一般很少有人吃韭菜。因为夏天韭菜多老化,纤维多而粗糙,不易被吸收。

Leeks are warm in nature, which can replenish kidney *qi* and invigorate energy. In spring, the body's liver *qi* is too exuberant, which would restrict the spleen(soil), so it will affect the transportation function of spleen and stomach. Eating leek can enhance the *qi* of spleen and stomach. But in summer, especially in June, few people eat leeks. Because leeks are aging in summer, and the fiber is too coarse to be easily absorbed.

----- 健康小提示 ------------------------------ **Health-preserving Tips**

韭菜不宜与白酒同食,易引起胃炎、溃疡病,易致肝病及出血性疾病。

Eating leeks and liquor together can easily cause gastritis, ulcers, liver disease and hemorrhagic disease.

13 五月鲤赛如活人参。
Carp in May is rich in nutrition.

鲤鱼是一种淡水鱼,营养成分非常丰富,富含大量的蛋白质、脂肪、钙离子、铁离子和多种游离的氨基酸,食之不但可以补充身体所需要的能量,还可以补充人体必需的维生素 A、维生素 B、维生素 C 和组织蛋白。

Carp is a freshwater fish with rich nutrients. It is rich in protein, fat, calcium ions, iron ions and a variety of free amino acids. Eating carp can not only supplement the energy needed by the body, but also replenish vitamin A, vitamin B, vitamin C and tissue protein that human beings need.

------ 健康小提示 ----------------------------- **Health-preserving Tips**

绿豆、芋头以及猪肝不能与鲤鱼同食,否则会引发腹痛或者腹泻等不良症状,对健康不利。

Mung beans, taro and pork liver should not be eaten with carp, otherwise it will cause adverse symptoms such as abdominal pain or diarrhea, which is harmful to health.

14 四季脾旺不受邪。
One is not easy to get sick if his/her spleen is healthy all year round.

脾对人体身体抵御邪气起着一定的防卫作用。脾的盛衰,关系到人体抗病能力的强弱。

The spleen helps people resist pathogenic *qi*. The functions of the spleen are related to the strength of people's ability to resist diseases.

------ 健康小提示 ----------------------------- **Health-preserving Tips**

每天上午九点到十一点要多喝水,让脾脏处于最活跃的状态;此时不宜食用燥热及辛辣刺激性的食物,以免伤胃败脾。

One should drink plenty of water from 9 a. m. to 11 a. m. every day to keep the spleen in its most active state; at this time, it is not advisable to eat hot and spicy food to avoid hurting the stomach and spleen.

15　药食同源。

Medicine and food share the same origin.

此谚语告诉我们,药物和食物本来是相通的,不仅服药可以治病养生,饮食调养也可达到同样的目的。这句谚语强调食物也有自身的功效和属性,因此,饮食要注意搭配。

This proverb tells us that medicine and food are interlinked. Curing and health-preserving can be achieved not only by taking medicine, but also by diet. It emphasizes that food has its own functions and attributes. Therefore, food should be carefully matched.

----- 健康小提示 ----------------------------------- **Health-preserving Tips**

每个人的体质都不一样,我们要根据自身情况来选择合适的食物。

Everyone's physique is different. Therefore, one should choose the right food according to his/her physique and health.

16　夏不坐木。

It is harmful to sit on wood in summer.

天气再热也不能过于贪图凉快,出汗降温有益健康。夏天气温高,湿度大,久置露天的木制长椅经过雨淋,太阳一晒,温度升高,会向外散发出湿热,人们坐在这样的木制长椅上容易患皮肤病、风湿和关节炎等。

No matter how hot the weather is, one can't be too greedy for coolness. Cooling down through sweating is good for health. Moreover, the temperature and the humidity of the air are high in summer. The wooden benches that have been placed in the open air for a long time are exposed to rain. When the sun appears, the temperature will rise, and the wooden benches will emit damp and heat. Sitting on such wooden benches can cause people to suffer from skin diseases, rheumatism and arthritis.

------ 健康小提示 --- **Health-preserving Tips**

夏天可以打开风扇、空调,借助这些电器保持室内空气的流通。

In summer, fans and air conditioners can be turned on to keep indoor air circulating.

17 夏日需清补,诸病皆能除。
Eating bland and nutritious food in summer can cure many diseases.

夏天的饮食应该以清补、健脾、祛暑化湿为原则,选择清淡滋阴的食物,如鲫鱼、虾、瘦肉、香菇、银耳、薏米等。高温季节,人体新陈代谢加快,容易缺乏各种维生素,可以多吃水果蔬菜,补充人体必需的维生素。

The diet in summer should be based on the principles of moistening, tonifying, fortifying the spleen, dispelling summer heat and resolving dampness. One can choose light and *yin*-nourishing food, such as crucian, shrimp, lean meat, mushrooms, white fungus, and barley. When the temperature is high, the body's metabolism speeds up. People are easily deficient in various vitamins. People can eat more fruit and vegetables to supplement vitamins that human beings need.

------ 健康小提示 --- **Health-preserving Tips**

石斛有滋阴生津、去火的作用,夏季适当食用石斛可以提高人体免疫力。

Shihu (dendrobium) has the functions of nourishing *yin* to engender fluid and removing internal heat. Proper consumption of *shihu* in summer can improve human immunity.

18 心静自然凉。
One will not feel hot when he/she is calm.

本谚语强调控制好自己的情绪就能适应环境。这一养生哲理,充分体现了祖国医学"形神合一"的辩证统一关系。心情烦躁、情绪波动容易引起呼吸加快、心率加速、血压升高、代谢加快,从而导致体温骤升,不利于身心健康。

This proverb emphasizes that one can adapt to the environment by controlling his/her emotions. This philosophy of health preservation fully embodies the dialectical unity of "the unity of body and spirit" in TCM. Irritability and mood swings can easily cause faster breathing, faster heart rate, higher blood pressure, and faster metabolism, resulting in a sudden rise in body temperature, which is not conducive to one's physical and mental health.

------ **健康小提示** ----------------------------------- **Health-preserving Tips**

如果脾气急躁,心烦意乱,易激动,就是在气候凉爽时,也难以克服燥热感。除此之外,养生保健还应正确处理主观意识与客观环境之间既相对立又相统一的矛盾关系。

If one is irritable, upset and agitated, it is difficult to overcome the hotness even when the climate is cool. In addition, it is also necessary to correctly handle the contradictory relationship between subjective consciousness and objective environment that is both opposed and unified when preserving health.

19　端午苋菜赛猪肝,六月苋菜金不换。
Eating more edible amaranth in summer is good for health.

苋菜具有清热解毒、增强体质的功效,它凉血散瘀、清肝解毒,对于湿热所致的赤白痢疾及肝火上炎所致的目赤目痛、咽喉红肿不利等均有一定的辅助治疗作用。除此之外,苋菜还能防止肌肉痉挛,维持正常的心肌活动。

Edible amaranth has the effects of clearing heat and relieving toxin, and strengthening physical fitness. It cools blood and dissipates stasis, clears the liver and detoxifies. It serves as an auxiliary treatment for red and white dysentery caused by damp heat and red eyes and eye pain caused by liver fire, red and swollen throat. In addition, edible amaranth can prevent muscle spasms and maintain normal cardiac activity.

----- **健康小提示** --------------------------------- **Health-preserving Tips**

苋菜其性寒凉,易伤阳气,故脾阳不振、脾虚便溏或慢性腹泻患者不宜多食。

Edible amaranth is cold in nature and easily hurts *yang qi*. Patients with devitalized spleen *yang*, loose stools and chronic diarrhea should not eat too much edible amaranth.

20 夏葫芦, 秋丝瓜。

Eating bottle gourds in summer and loofah in autumn is good for health.

葫芦含有蛋白质及多种微量元素,有利于增强人体的免疫力,清热解毒也是它的一大功效,常吃葫芦可有效防治痤疮,在夏季食用有利健康。丝瓜是日常生活中比较常见的一种蔬菜,具有清热利湿、凉血解毒的功效。秋天适量地吃一些丝瓜可以有效消退因肺热导致的咳嗽和上火现象。

Bottle gourd contains protein and a variety of trace elements, which is beneficial to enhance the our immunity. Clearing heat and relieving toxin are also its major effects. Eating bottle gourds often can prevent acne effectively, which is very suitable for consumption in summer. Loofah is a common vegetable. It has the effects of clearing heat and draining damp, and cooling the blood and detoxification. Eating loofah in an appropriate amount in autumn can effectively relieve the cough and fire caused by lung heat.

----- **健康小提示** --------------------------------- **Health-preserving Tips**

腹泻患者不宜吃丝瓜,因为丝瓜性寒,并且含有大量可以促进肠胃消化的膳食纤维。

Patients with diarrhea should not eat loofah because it is cold in nature and contains a lot of dietary fiber that can promote digestion.

21　原汤化原食。

Original soup helps people digest food.

中国饮食传统中,一直就有"原汤化原食"的说法。老人们在吃完捞面、水饺后,都要喝点原汤。这句谚语告诉我们,煮制淀粉类食品的汤有促进消化的作用,喝"原汤"有利于全面吸收食物中的营养成分。

In Chinese food traditions, there has always been a saying that "Original soup helps people digest food". Old people always drink some original soup after eating noodles and dumplings. This proverb tells us that the leftover soup from cooking starchy foods has the effect of promoting digestion, and drinking "original soup" is beneficial for one to fully absorb the nutrients in the food.

----- 健康小提示 ----------------------------- **Health-preserving Tips**

煮饺子的汤和面汤可以饮用。但是,火锅的汤则不同,因为火锅汤中油脂含量太高,有害健康。

Dumpling soup and noodle soup can be consumed. However, hot pot soup is different from them, because hot pot soup contains a lot of fat, which is harmful to health.

22　食不厌杂。

Diversity of food is good for health.

这句谚语是指人们的膳食应当广泛一些,粗粮、细粮、肉类、禽蛋、奶类、蔬菜、水果合理搭配,都要吃,这样才能健康。此谚语强调饮食营养要全面,这样才有益于健康。人是杂食动物,许多必需的营养元素自身无法合成。因此,摄取尽可能多种类的食物是我们的最好选择。

This proverb means that people should eat a wide range of food, such as coarse grains, fine grains, meat, eggs, milk, vegetables and fruit. It is emphasized that the nutrition of diet should be comprehensive, which is beneficial to health. People are omnivores, and many of necessary nutrients cannot be synthesized by themselves. Therefore, it is people's best choice to eat as many kinds of food as possible.

虽说食不厌杂,但是如果得了某些疾病需要忌口就是另外一回事了。例如,高血压患者和肾病患者要少吃盐,动脉硬化患者不能食用动物脂肪等。

Although one should eat a variety of food, he/she still needs to avoid certain food if he/she is sick. For example, patients with hypertension and kidney disease should eat less salt, and patients with arteriosclerosis should not eat animal fat.

23 荷叶茯苓粥,利五脏通经络。

Porridge made with lotus leaves and *fuling* (Indian bread) can benefit the five *zang* viscera and dredge meridian and collateral.

中医认为荷叶具有清热利湿、解毒化痰、凉血止血的作用。茯苓是寄生在松树根上的一种真菌,其药用价值很高,能全方位地增强人体的免疫功能,是老年人延年益寿的良药。茯苓安神、健脾和胃、利水渗湿。炎热的夏季用荷叶和茯苓搭配煮粥,食之不但清香甘甜,对五脏也有保健作用。

TCM believes that lotus leaves have the functions of clearing heat and draining damp, detoxification, resolving phlegm, cooling blood and stopping bleeding. *Fuling* is a kind of fungus parasitic on the roots of pine trees. It has high medicinal value and can enhance the immune function of human body in an all-round way. It is a good medicine for the old to prolong their lives. *Fuling* has the functions of tranquilizing, invigorating spleen and harmonizing stomach, inducing diuresis and draining damp. One can put lotus leaf and *fuling* together to make porridge in summer. It is not only fragrant and sweet, but also has a healthy effect on the five *zang* viscera.

体瘦气血虚弱者最好不要服用荷叶,气虚者忌服茯苓。茯苓会阻碍人体生长发育,儿童和青少年不宜食用。

People who are thin and weak in *qi* and blood had better not eat lotus leaves. *Fuling* should not be taken by the patients with deficiency *qi*. *Fuling* can hinder the growth and development of the human body, so it is not suitable for children and adolescents to eat.

24　十苦九补数苦瓜。

Most bitter foods can replenish the body, and bitter gourds rank the first.

苦瓜含有类胰岛素活性物质及多种氨基酸,具有明显的降血糖作用,被称为"植物胰岛素",对糖尿病有一定疗效。多吃苦瓜使女性身材苗条纤美,皮肤滋润光洁、细嫩白皙。苦瓜的维生素 C 含量很高,还有一定的抗病毒能力。

Bitter gourd contains insulin-like active substances and a variety of amino acids, which has obvious hypoglycemic effect, so it is known as "plant insulin", and it has curative effect on diabetes. Eating more bitter gourds can make women slim and beautiful, and their skin will be moist, smooth and white. The vitamin C content of bitter gourds is very high, which has antiviral ability.

----- **健康小提示** ----------------------------- **Health-preserving Tips**

从超市买苦瓜干用热水冲泡当茶喝是不错的选择,但是脾胃虚弱者不宜食用。

It's a good choice to buy dried bitter gourds from the supermarket and brew it with hot water as tea, but it's not suitable for people with asthenia of spleen and stomach.

25　三伏不离绿豆汤,头顶火盆身无恙。

Drinking mung bean soup in dog days will not be uncomfortable even if the brazier is overhead.

绿豆含有丰富的矿物质和维生素。此外,绿豆还具有解暑功效,在炎热的三伏天,适当喝一些绿豆汤不仅能够补充身体缺少的矿物质,还可以调节机体水盐

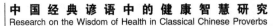
代谢平衡。

Mung beans are rich in minerals and vitamins. In addition, mung beans also have the effect of releasing summer heat. In the hot summer days, drinking some mung bean soup can not only replenish minerals for people, but also regulate water and salt metabolism balance of the body.

------ 健康小提示 ------------------------------- **Health-preserving Tips**

中医认为,绿豆性寒,空腹饮用容易伤脾胃。

TCM believes that mung beans are cold in nature. Drinking mung bean soup on an empty stomach can easily hurt the spleen and the stomach.

26 杨梅开胃祛暑热。

Bayberries can increase appetite and relieve summer heat.

新鲜的杨梅是夏季祛暑的水果佳品。杨梅含有多种有机酸,维生素 C 的含量也十分丰富,鲜果味酸,使用以后可增加胃中酸度,有助于消化食物,增进食欲。

Fresh bayberry is a good fruit for releasing summer heat. Bayberries contain vitamin C and a variety of organic acids. The fresh bayberries taste sour. Eating bayberries can help to increase acidity in the stomach, digest food, and promote appetite.

------ 健康小提示 ------------------------------- **Health-preserving Tips**

吃杨梅前最好用盐水浸泡几分钟,这样可以洗掉一些脏东西,还可使杨梅的风味更佳。

One should soak bayberries in salt water for a few minutes before eating them. This method can wash away the dirty things on the surface of the bayberries and make the bayberries more delicious.

第三节　秋季养生
Section Three　Health Preserving in Autumn

1　秋日甘蔗赛过参。
Sugarcane in autumn is more nutritious than ginseng.

秋天的甘蔗水分充足,营养丰富。多吃甘蔗能够滋阴润燥,尤其是能缓解秋燥引起的水分缺失和心理烦躁现象。在为身体补充水分的同时,甘蔗还可以保持皮肤的滋润与光泽,安神去火。

Sugarcane in autumn is rich in water and nutrition. Eating more sugarcane can nourish *yin* and moisten dryness, especially relieve the phenomenon of water deficiency and psychological irritability caused by dryness in autumn. While replenishing water for the body, sugarcane can also keep the skin moist and glossy, calm the nerves and reduce internal heat.

------ 健康小提示 ----------------------------- **Health-preserving Tips**

咳嗽痰少或者胃液分泌不足的人应该多吃甘蔗。此外,多吃甘蔗可以预防便秘。

People who cough with less sputum or lack of gastric juice should eat more sugarcane. In addition, eating more sugarcane can prevent constipation.

2　四季不离蒜,不用去医院。
Eating garlic all year round keeps the doctor away.

大蒜是日常生活中常用的调味品,在中医药学中,它也是十分适宜常年食用的养生之物。经常食用可提高身体免疫力,增加抗病性。

Garlic is a condiment commonly used in daily life. In TCM, it is also a health preserving food suitable for perennial consumption. Eating garlic often can improve one's immunity and disease resistance ability.

空腹不要吃大蒜,大蒜比较辛辣,容易刺激肠胃,有可能引起肠胃炎。

Don't eat garlic on an empty stomach. Garlic is spicy, which can easily stimulate the stomach and cause gastroenteritis.

3 青菜萝卜糙米饭,瓦壶天水菊花茶。

Natural foods such as vegetables, radish, brown rice and chrysanthemum tea are good for health.

多吃青菜不但可补充防癌的叶酸,还可以缓解便秘,预防大肠癌。萝卜有消食、化痰定喘的功能。常吃糙米能够促进血液循环,降低脂肪和胆固醇。菊花茶具有散热功效,可治疗因肺热所致的发热、咳嗽、头痛等症状。

Eating more green vegetables can not only supplement folic acid, but also relieve constipation and prevent colorectal cancer. Radish has the functions of promoting digestion, and resolving phlegm and asthma. Eating brown rice often can promote blood circulation and reduce fat and cholesterol. Chrysanthemum tea has the effect of dissipating heat. It can treat fever, cough, headache and other symptoms caused by lung heat.

脾胃虚弱者最好不要喝菊花茶。

People with asthenia of spleen and stomach had better not drink chrysanthemum tea.

4 立了秋,把扇丢。

One won't need a fan after autumn begins.

立秋之后天气转凉,不需要摇扇纳凉了。立秋是二十四节气中第十三个节气,于公历8月7日至9日交节。立秋是秋季的第一个节气,为秋季的起点。进入秋季以后,万物开始从茂盛走向萧索。

The weather turns cool after the beginning of autumn, so there's no need to shake the fan. The beginning of autumn is the 13th solar term of the 24 solar terms. It is held from August 7 to 9 of the Gregorian calendar. The beginning of autumn is the first solar term of autumn, which is the starting point of autumn. In autumn, everything begins to move from luxuriant to bleak.

------ **健康小提示** ------------------------------ **Health-preserving Tips**

老年人对秋天气候变化的适应性和耐受力较差,更应重视预防疾病。

The old people's adaptability and tolerance to climate change in autumn are weak, so they should pay more attention to the prevention of diseases.

5　金秋欲解燥,梨子百合最奇妙。

Pears and *baihe* (lily) can relieve dryness in autumn.

中医理论认为:秋天与人体肺脏相应,故燥气易入肺经,许多人到了秋天就咽部不适,这是秋燥所致。生吃梨能明显解除此症状。常食百合有润肺止咳、养心安神、健脾和胃之效。

According to the theory of TCM, autumn corresponds to the lung, so dryness is easy to enter the lung channel. Many people get throat discomfort in autumn. It is caused by "autumn dryness". Eating raw pears can obviously relieve the symptom. Eating *baihe* (lily) often can moisten lung and stop cough, nourish the heart and calm the nerves, invigorate spleen and harmonize stomach.

------ **健康小提示** ------------------------------ **Health-preserving Tips**

脾胃虚寒者不要吃梨。梨中糖分较高,糖尿病患者不宜食用。

People with asthenia of spleen and stomach should not eat pears. Pears are rich in sugar, so they are not suitable for diabetics.

6 柑橘营养价值高,理气健脾润秋燥。

Citrus is rich in nutrients, which can regulate *qi* and invigorate the spleen.

柑橘具有理气解郁、止咳化痰的作用。从营养学的角度来讲,柑橘中的维生素 C、维生素 B、维生素 E 等含量非常丰富,可以有效地滋养神经,消除颜面部位的色素沉着、对抗氧化,并且可以降低血压、血脂。

Citrus has the functions of regulating *qi*, relieving depression, suppressing cough and resolving phlegm. From the perspective of nutrition, citrus is rich in vitamin C, vitamin B and vitamin E, which can effectively nourish nerves, eliminate facial pigmentation, resist oxidation, and reduce blood pressure and blood lipid.

----- 健康小提示 ----------------------------- **Health-preserving Tips**

柑橘类水果内都有一层"白丝","白丝"中含有比较多的纤维素和多酚类物质,具有一定的抗氧化抗衰老作用,所以吃柑橘时最好带着"白丝"一起吃。

There is a layer of "white silk" in citrus fruits, which contains cellulose and polyphenols, and has anti-oxidation and anti-aging effect, so one had better eat citrus with "white silk".

7 金秋防秋乏。

One should prevent autumn weariness in autumn.

入秋以后,人的身体进入休整阶段。秋乏是机体恢复体力的保护性措施,补偿盛夏给人体带来的过度消耗。

The human body is in the rest stage in autumn. Autumn weariness is a protective measure to recover the body's physical strength, which compensates for the excessive consumption brought by midsummer.

----- 健康小提示 ----------------------------- **Health-preserving Tips**

要缓解秋乏,人们要注意饮食,加强营养,劳逸结合,最好多出门做运动,呼

吸新鲜空气。

In order to alleviate autumn weariness, people should attach importance to rational diet, supplement nutrition and balance work and rest. It's better for them to go out and do more exercise and breathe fresh air.

8 入秋食板栗，健胃又补脾。

Eating chestnuts in autumn helps us invigorate stomach and spleen.

板栗营养成分非常丰富，含有大量蛋白质、淀粉、维生素 A、胡萝卜素及矿物质等，除了鲜美软糯的口感外，还具有养胃、健脾、补肾、补充维生素等功效。

Chestnut is rich in nutrients, including protein, starch, vitamin A, carotene and minerals. In addition to the delicious taste of soft waxy, it also has the functions of nourishing stomach, strengthening spleen, tonifying kidney and supplementing vitamins.

----- 健康小提示 ----------------------------- **Health-preserving Tips**

板栗和羊肉二者都不易消化，同时食用这两种食物很容易引起呕吐。

Chestnuts and mutton are not easy to digest, and eating both of them at the same time can easily cause vomiting.

9 秋里萝卜抵过肉。

Eating radish in autumn is healthier than eating meat.

秋天吃萝卜，不仅能润肺降燥，还能滋养咽喉，有效预防感冒。萝卜中含有的芥子油，可以有效促进肠胃蠕动，增强消化能力，增加食欲，对人体大有益处，所以说"秋里萝卜抵过肉"。

Eating radish in autumn can not only moisturize the lungs and reduce dryness, but also nourish the throat and prevent colds effectively. The mustard oil contained in radish can promote gastrointestinal motility, enhance digestion and increase the appetite effectively, and it is beneficial to the health. Therefore, it is said that "Eating radish in autumn is healthier than eating meat."

萝卜和橘子不能同时吃,否则会导致甲状腺肿大。

Radishes and oranges can not be eaten together, otherwise it will lead to goiter.

10 吃了十月茄,饿死郎中爷。

Eating eggplant in October makes one's doctor a beggar.

茄子是人们在日常餐桌上常吃的一种蔬菜,它不仅味道好、营养丰富,还具有防病治病的功效。中医认为,茄子味甘、性苦寒,有散血淤、治疗寒热、通风活络和止血等多种功效,可有效治疗内痔、大便出血、皮肤溃烂、风热湿疹等病症。

Eggplant is a kind of vegetable that people often eat in daily life. It not only has good taste and rich nutrition, but also has the effect of disease prevention and treatment. According to TCM, eggplant is sweet in taste and bitter in nature. It has many functions, such as dispersing blood stasis, treating cold and heat, ventilating and activating collaterals and stopping the bleeding. It can effectively treat internal hemorrhoids, stool bleeding, skin ulceration, wind heat eczema and other diseases.

茄子含有丰富的花青素,有美容养颜之功效,但茄子性凉,所以脾胃虚寒、腹泻、消化不良者不宜多食。

Eggplant is rich in anthocyanins, which has the effect of beautifying. However, eggplant is cool in nature, so people with asthenia of spleen and stomach, diarrhea, and indigestion should not eat more.

11 十月火旺旺,多喝芥菜汤。

Drinking leaf mustard soup in October can help reduce internal heat.

芥菜汤是以芥菜为主要原料,煮制而成的一道家常菜。芥菜的营养成分十分丰富,含有大量的膳食纤维,胡萝卜素,维生素 C,钙、镁、钠、磷等微量元素和碳水化合物。经常服用芥菜汤,有助于消肿解毒、明目、提神醒脑。

Leaf mustard soup is a home cooked dish with leaf mustard as the main raw material. Leaf mustard is rich in nutrients, including a lot of dietary fiber, carotene, vitamin C, calcium, magnesium, sodium, phosphorus and other trace elements and carbohydrates. Taking leaf mustard soup often can help us relieve swelling and detoxification, improve eyesight and refresh the brain.

------ **健康小提示** ----------------------------------- **Health-preserving Tips**

芥菜汤不能过多食用。芥菜性温,长期喝芥菜汤会引发痔疮,或导致肝脏受损。

One should not consume too much leaf mustard soup. Leaf mustard is warm in nature. Long-term consumption of leaf mustard soup can cause hemorrhoids and liver damage.

第四节 冬季养生
Section Four Health Preserving in Winter

1 冬天先护脚,病魔不来找。
One can warm feet in winter to avoid illness.

脚处于人体最下端,血液供应比其他部位少,且表面脂肪薄,不易保暖。中医有"寒从足下生"的说法。疾病和季节是有一定联系的。进入冬季以后,天气寒冷,空气干燥,年轻人容易受凉感冒,老年人的一些旧病(如支气管炎、哮喘等)容易复发。脚部有很多穴位,且人体有 6 条脉络系于脚部。泡脚可促进血液循环,驱逐脚部寒气,增强人体免疫力。

The feet are at the bottom of the human body, and the blood supply is less than other parts, and the surface fat is thin, which makes it difficult for them to keep warm. There is a saying in TCM that "Cold is born from feet. " There is a certain connection between disease and season. After entering the winter, the weather is cold and the air is dry. Young people are prone to catch colds. Some chronic diseases of the elderly (such as bronchitis, asthma, etc.) are easy to relapse. There are many acupoints on the feet, and the human body has six meridians hidden in the feet. Feet soaking can promote blood circulation, expel the cold of the feet and enhance human immunity.

----- 健康小提示 ---------------------------- Health-preserving Tips

热水能使血管扩张、血流加快。每天用合适温度的热水泡脚,不仅可以加速血液循环,还可以滋润脚部皮肤,达到缓解疲劳的功效。

Hot water can dilate blood vessels and speed up blood flow. Soaking feet with hot water at the right temperature every day can not only speed up blood circulation, but also moisturize the skin of the feet to relieve fatigue.

2　冬天动一动,少闹一场病。
Exercise more in winter to avoid illness.

冬天人体不断受到冷空气的刺激,人体造血机能也发生变化。血液中的红细胞、白细胞、白蛋白及抵抗疾病的抗体增多,从而大大提高了人体对疾病的抵抗力,有助于预防感冒、气管炎、贫血和肺炎。冬天到户外参加体育活动,身体受到寒冷的刺激,肌肉、血管不停地收缩,能够促使心跳加快,呼吸加深,体内新陈代谢加强,身体产生的热量增加。同时,由于大脑皮质兴奋性增强,体温调节中枢的能力明显提高,这样,就会增强人的抗寒能力。

In winter, the human body is constantly stimulated by the cold air, and the human hematopoietic function also changes. The increase of red blood cells, white blood cells, albumin and antibodies against diseases in the blood greatly improves the body's resistance to diseases and helps prevent colds, bronchitis, anemia and pneumonia. When participating in sports activities outdoors in winter, the body is stimulated by the cold. Muscles and blood vessels keep contracting, which can speed up the heart rate, deepen breathing, strengthen the metabolism and increase the heat of body. At the same time, due to the increased excitability of the cerebral cortex, the ability of the body temperature regulation center is significantly improved, which will enhance people's ability to resist the cold.

健康小提示 ------------------------------------ **Health-preserving Tips**

冬季户外锻炼时也要补充水分,可以饮用普通的水或运动饮料,但热咖啡或巧克力不是好的选择,反而会造成人体失水。

One should drink water during outdoor exercise in winter. One can drink ordinary water or sports drinks. Hot coffee and chocolate are not good choices because they will lead to water loss.

3　冬天一碗姜糖汤,去风去寒赛仙方。

Ginger sugar soup can drive away the wind and the cold in winter.

姜汤祛湿寒、温热,适合体质虚寒的人饮用。姜汤还能润肺止燥、杀菌灭菌、舒筋活血。女性多喝红糖水可以缓解痛经。姜与红糖一起煮对人体有温和调理的功效。

Ginger soup dispels dampness and cold, and it is suitable for people with weak and cold constitution. Ginger soup can also moisten the lungs, relieve dryness, sterilize, and relax muscles and blood. Women can drink more brown sugar water to relieve dysmenorrhea. Cooking ginger and brown sugar together has a gentle conditioning effect on the human body.

健康小提示 ------------------------------------ **Health-preserving Tips**

生姜味道辛辣,使人振奋,所以最好不要在晚上喝姜糖汤,否则会影响人的正常入睡。

The fresh ginger tastes spicy and makes people excited. People should not drink ginger sugar soup at night, otherwise it will affect normal sleep.

4　红枣芹菜根,能降胆固醇。

Chinese red dates and celery root can lower cholesterol.

红枣具有一定的补益脾胃、滋养阴血、养心安神等功效,对记忆力减退、阿尔茨海默病、胆固醇增高等病症有辅助治疗作用。芹菜是高纤维食物,能够抑制肠内致癌物质的生产,加快粪便排泄,预防大肠癌。平时多吃红枣和芹菜有益健康。

Chinese red dates have the effects of nourishing spleen and stomach, supplementing *yin*-blood, nourishing the heart and inducing tranquilization. It has an adjuvant therapeutic effect on memory loss, Alzheimer's disease, and elevated cholesterol. Celery is a high-fiber food that can inhibit the production of carcinogens in the intestines, speed up fecal excretion, and prevent colorectal cancer. Eating more Chinese red dates and celery is good for health.

----- 健康小提示 ----------------------------- **Health-preserving Tips**

芹菜性凉,大便溏泻的人不宜多食。另外,芹菜有降血压作用,所以血压偏低的人要慎食。

Celery is cold in nature. People who are prone to diarrhea should not eat it. In addition, celery has the effect of lowering blood pressure, so people with low blood pressure had better not eat celery.

5 红枣黄芪汤,补血养气好效方。

Chinese red dates and *huangqi* (milkvetch root) decoction are effective in nourishing blood and *qi*.

红枣富含维生素、果糖和各种氨基酸。中医认为红枣性暖、养血保血,能够改善血液循环。气血两虚、脾胃功能不好的人可以多吃。黄芪也是用来补气血的食物,在做菜的时候适当加入一些可以起到养生保健的作用,还能加强食疗的效果。

Chinese red dates are rich in vitamins, fructose and various amino acids. TCM believes that Chinese red dates are warm in nature, can nourish and protect blood and improve blood circulation. People with deficiency of both *qi* and blood and asthenia of spleen and stomach had better eat more Chinese red dates. *Huangqi* is also used to replenish *qi* and blood. Adding some *huangqi* properly in the food can not only keep healthy, but also strengthen the effect of dietotherapy.

----- 健康小提示 ----------------------------- **Health-preserving Tips**

黄芪性温,所以有便秘、热毒、发烧、咳血、阳亢的人士不宜食用。

Huangqi is warm in nature, so it is not suitable for people with constipation, heat toxin, fever, hemoptysis and hyperactivity of *yang*.

6 冬季多晒太阳,有利健康。

Bathing in the sun in winter is good for health.

冬天晒太阳,和大自然进行接触,可以提高人体血液循环速度,调节神经中枢。每天晒太阳一小时左右,有利于身体健康,适量的阳光照射会使人感到舒适,起到活血化瘀的作用。

Bathing in the sun in winter can improve the blood circulation speed of the human body, regulate the nerve center. Basking in the sun for about an hour every day is conducive to health. An appropriate amount of sunlight will make people feel comfortable and play the role of activating blood and resolving stasis.

----- 健康小提示 ----------------------------- **Health-preserving Tips**

虽然冬季的阳光不如夏季的强烈,但还是会对眼睛造成很大的伤害,所以晒太阳的时候别忘了戴上墨镜或者遮阳帽。

Although the sunlight in winter is not as strong as that in summer, it still does great harm to the eyes. So don't forget to wear sunglasses or sunshade hat when basking in the sun.

7 冬吃萝卜夏吃姜,不劳医生开药方。

Radishes in winter and ginger in summer makes the doctor an idler.

冬季,天气寒冷,人体皮肤腠理处于收缩状态,以保证身体的血液供应。而这个阶段,人的户外活动减少,室内活动增加,而且很多人进食大量热性食物,容易产生内热,从而引起消化不良,这个时候吃一些萝卜可以帮助消化。夏天炎热,人体为了排除体内的热量,皮肤腠理处于开放的状态,热量容易散失,而这个时候吃一些姜有助于暖胃,可达到身体阴阳平衡的目的。

The weather is cold in winter, and the skin is in a state of contraction to ensure the blood supply of the body. At this stage, people's outdoor activities decrease, indoor activities increase, and most of them eat a lot of hot food, which is easy to produce internal heat and cause indigestion. Eating some radishes at this time can help improve the digesting function. It's hot in summer. In order to eliminate the heat in the body, the skin is in an open state, and the heat is easy to be dissipated. At this time, eating some ginger will help to warm the stomach and balance *yin* and *yang* of the body.

----- 健康小提示 ------------------------------- Health-preserving Tips

白萝卜富含维生素 C,对人体健康非常有益,而若与胡萝卜混合就会使维生素 C 丧失殆尽。因为胡萝卜中含有一种抗坏血酸的解酵素,此物质会破坏白萝卜中的维生素 C。

White radish is rich in vitamin C, which is very beneficial to human health. If it is mixed with carrot, vitamin C will be lost because carrots contain an enzyme called ascorbic acid, which can destroy vitamin C in white radish.

8 冬补三九,夏补三伏。
One should nourish the body during the coldest and hottest times.

中医认为,冬令进补与平衡阴阳、疏通经络以及调和气血关系密切。在寒冷的冬季,老年人抵抗能力降低,更应该进行食补,以获得药物所不能替代的效果。夏季昼长夜短,人体精力损耗大,体重下降快,此时进补比较容易吸收,可以防止虚衰。

TCM believes that tonic in winter is closely related to balancing *yin* and *yang*, freeing the channels and networks vessels and regulating *qi* and blood. In the cold winter, the elderly's resistance is reduced, so they should take tonic food, which shows the effect that medicine can't replace. In summer, the days are long and the nights are short, and people consume a lot of energy and lose weight quickly. At this time, it is easier for people to absorb nutrients, which can prevent decay.

----- 健康小提示 ------------------------- **Health-preserving Tips**

夏季滋补与冬季滋补不同,一定要清淡,不可过于滋养油腻,否则容易伤胃。

One should follow different principles to supplement the body in summer and winter. In summer, one should eat light tonics, otherwise the stomach may be hurt.

9 冬令进补,开春打虎。

One who takes tonics in winter is strong enough to fight a tiger in spring.

冬季的气候特点为"寒",中医学认为,寒为阴邪,人体受外界影响,阴气也相应增加,伤及人体的阳气,此时人体为抵御严寒,需要储存更多的能量和营养物质。因此,冬季是人体进补的最佳时节。

The climate in winter is characterized by "cold". According to TCM, cold is *yin* pathogen. Affected by the outside environment, *yin qi* increases correspondingly, damaging *yang qi*. At this time, the human body needs to store more energy and nutrients to resist the cold. Therefore, winter is the best time to nourish the body.

----- 健康小提示 ------------------------- **Health-preserving Tips**

一般而言,在冬季,中青年人以补益脾胃为主,老年人以补益肾气为主。对于脾胃消化不良的人来说,首先要恢复脾胃的功能,否则服再多的补物也是无用。

Generally speaking, in winter, the young people mainly tonify the spleen and the stomach, and the old mainly tonify the kidney *qi*. For people with indigestion of spleen and stomach, the first thing to do is to restore the function of spleen and stomach, otherwise it is useless to take supplements.

10　冬令进补秋垫底。

Conditioning the body in autumn is good for nourishing the body in winter.

冬天想要补好,需要提前调理好身体。否则,身体不仅难以吸收补品的营养,还会事与愿违地被其所伤,引发湿热加重等问题。

If one wants to nourish his/her body in winter, he/she needs to adjust his/her body in advance. Otherwise, the body will not only be difficult to absorb the nutrition of supplements, but also be hurt by them resulting in the aggravation of damp heat and other problems.

------ 健康小提示 ----------------------------- **Health-preserving Tips**

一般人不用刻意进补,药补不如食补,好好吃饭,加强锻炼,就能增强体质。如果确实虚弱需要进补,一定要咨询正规医院的医生,辨证论治。一旦出现流鼻血、口腔溃疡、大便秘结等问题要立即停止进补。

People in general don't need to take tonics studiously. It's better to take tonics than medicine. Reasonable diet and exercise can enhance the physique. If one is really weak and needs tonics, he/she must consult a doctor in a regular hospital and follow the principle of syndrome differentiation and treatment. If there is nosebleed, oral ulcer, constipation and other problems, one should stop tonics immediately.

11　冬病夏治,重在预防。

Diseases that may be caught in winter should be treated in summer and prevention should be the priority.

"冬病夏治"是中医上一个极具特色的重要方法。夏季气温高,人体阳气充沛,体表经络中气血旺盛,用药物来调整人体的阴阳平衡,可以治愈一些疾病。可以说,"冬病夏治"体现了中医学中人与自然相协调的整体观念和预防为主的理念。

"Diseases that may be caught in winter should be treated in summer" is an important method with great characteristics in TCM. The temperature is high in summer, the body is full of *yang qi*, and the meridians on the body surface are full of *qi* and blood. Using medicine to balance *yin* and *yang* can cure some diseases. It can be said that "Diseases that may be caught in winter should be treated in summer" embodies the holistic concept of harmony between man and nature in TCM and the concept of focusing on disease prevention.

----- **健康小提示** ----------------------------- **Health-preserving Tips**

对于哮喘病、慢性支气管炎、过敏性鼻炎等慢性呼吸道疾病患者,"冬病夏治"能起到调节免疫、改善肺功能、平喘止咳的效果。

For patients with asthma, chronic bronchitis, allergic rhinitis and other chronic respiratory diseases, "Diseases that may be caught in winter should be treated in summer" can regulate immunity, improve lung function and relieve asthma and cough.

12 冬天要吃"黑"。
Eat food with black outer color in winter is good for health.

中医"五行养生"理论认为,冬季五行属水,人体五脏中属水的为肾。因此,冬季养生补肾,会有事半功倍的效果。黑色属肾,补肾要多吃黑色食物。

According to the theory of "five elements of health preserving" in TCM, the five elements in winter belong to water, and the water in the five *zang* viscera is the kidney. Therefore, tonifying kidney in winter helps to keep healthy. TCM holds that black and kidney are related, and eating more black food can tonify the kidney.

----- **健康小提示** ----------------------------- **Health-preserving Tips**

传统中医学认为,黑豆有助于抗衰老,具有医食同疗的特殊功能,含较丰富的蛋白质、脂肪、碳水化合物、胡萝卜素、维生素、烟酸等营养物质,所含的雌激素有助于延缓衰老,养颜美容。黑豆还有益于治疗水肿,且活血解毒。药理研究结果显示,黑豆能养阴补气。

According to TCM, black bean is helpful to anti-aging and has the special function of treating medicine and food together. It is rich in protein, fat, carbohydrate, carotene, vitamin, niacin and other nutrients, and its estrogen helps to delay aging and nourish beauty. Black beans help to treat edema, promote blood circulation and detoxify. Pharmacological research results show that black beans can nourish *yin qi*.

13　冬季戴棉帽，如同穿棉袄。

Wearing a thick hat in winter is as warm as wearing a wadded jacket.

寒冷的冬天，人们一般都会穿上棉服御寒，但是却很少有人重视头部的保暖。人的头部是大脑神经中枢的所在地，头部的皮肤很薄，但血管粗，汗毛多，所以体内热能的散发量也很大。体热从头部散发出去后，人体内的阳气便会受损。

In the cold winter, people usually wear cotton padded clothes to keep warm, but few people attach importance to the warmth of the head. The nerve center of brain is in the head. The skin of the head is very thin, but the blood vessels are thick and there are many sweat hairs, so there's a lot of heat coming out of the body. When the heat is emitted from the head, *yang qi* in the body will be damaged.

----- 健康小提示 ----------------------------- Health-preserving Tips

冬季戴帽应特别注重让帽子护住耳朵。老年人由于自主神经功能下降，基础代谢率低，防寒能力差，更要时时都戴帽子。

One should protect the ears when wearing the hat in winter. Due to the decline of autonomic nervous function, low basal metabolic rate and poor cold resistance, the elderly should always wear hats.

14　冬伤于寒，春必病温。

If people are seriously injured by cold pathogen in winter, they will get sick in the spring of the next year.

如果人们在冬天受到寒邪的严重伤害，到来年春天会生病。中医认为，四季的特点分别为春生、夏长、秋收、冬藏。冬季的到来,会使阳气潜藏、阴气盛极,万物活动也都趋向休止,纷纷养精蓄锐,为来年春天的生机勃发做好储备。人也同样要顺应大自然,藏精纳气,保存体力,增强自身的免疫力。这样,在来年春天万物复苏,各种病菌蠢蠢欲动时,才能更好地抵御它们的侵袭。

If people are seriously injured by cold pathogen in winter, they will get sick in the spring of the next year. TCM believes that the characteristics of the four seasons are birth, growth, harvest and storage. The arrival of winter will make *yang qi* hidden and *yin qi* excessive. All activities will tend to stop and replenish energy for the vitality in the next spring. Humans also have to conform to nature, store essence and absorb *qi* to preserve physical strength and enhance their own immunity. In this way, when everything recovers in the coming spring and various germs are ready to move, people can better resist their invasion.

------ 健康小提示 ---------------------------------- Health-preserving Tips

只有在冬天把阳气补足了,才能拥有强壮的身躯去抵抗病邪。

Only when the body is supplemented with *yang qi* in the winter, will one have a strong body to resist diseases in the coming year.

15　冬不蒙首,春不露背。

Don't cover the head when sleeping in winter; don't leave the back naked when sleeping in spring.

天冷的时候不要蒙头睡,因为被子里的空气不循环,人体呼出的二氧化碳容易在厚被子中积聚,造成体内缺氧。天气开始转暖的时候不要掀开被子露出背部。中医认为"背为阳",阳气被外界吸收以后容易引发督脉病痛,诸如腰背疼痛、风湿性关节炎等。

Don't sleep with the head covered in winter because the air in the quilt does not circulate, and the carbon dioxide exhaled by the human body tends to accumulate in the thick quilt, causing hypoxia. Don't lift the quilt to expose the back when the it starts to warm. TCM believes that "The attribute of the back is *yang*." The absorption of *yang qi* by the outside world may lead to governor vessel diseases, such as low back pain and rheumatoid arthritis.

----- 健康小提示 ----------------------------- **Health-preserving Tips**

冬天睡觉盖被子的同时一定要露出头部,让鼻腔顺利呼吸。肩胛骨要盖好,避免因风寒而患肩周炎、感冒。

When sleeping under the quilt in winter, one must expose his/her head to breathe smoothly. The scapula should be covered well to avoid suffering from scapulohumeral periarthritis and cold due to wind cold.

16 冬吃羊肉夏吃鸭,不冷不热吃鲜鱼。

Eat lamb in winter; eat duck in summer; eat fish when the temperature is comfortable.

羊肉富含蛋白质、维生素以及多种微量元素。寒冬吃羊肉可益气补虚、促进血液循环、增强御寒能力、提高身体免疫力。夏季吃鸭肉可以补充丰富的水分,防止因为出汗过多而形成脱水现象。中医认为,鸭肉可以补中益气、健脾开胃,对于气血亏虚导致的头晕头痛、脾胃虚弱和食欲不振有很好的调节作用。鱼类中含有丰富的 DHA 和卵磷脂,可以提高人的记忆力。

Mutton is rich in protein, vitamins and a variety of trace elements. Eating mutton in the cold winter can replenish *qi*, promote blood circulation, enhance cold resistance and improve immunity. Eating duck meat in summer can replenish water and prevent dehydration due to excessive sweating. TCM holds that duck meat can invigorate spleen-stomach and replenish *qi*. What's more, it has regulating effect on dizziness, headache, asthenia of spleen and stomach and loss of appetite caused by deficiency of *qi* and blood. Fish is rich in DHA and lecithin, which can improve our memory.

----- 健康小提示 ----------------------------- **Health-preserving Tips**

经常口腔溃疡、眼睛红、口苦、烦躁、咽喉干痛、齿龈肿痛者及腹泻者均不宜多食羊肉和鸭肉。

People who are prone to oral ulcer, red eyes, bitter mouth, irritability, sore dry throat, sore gums, and diarrhea had better not eat lamb or duck.

17　冬至饺子夏至面。

Eat dumplings at the winter solstice and noodles at the summer solstice.

夏至食面,"面"一般指的是面条。因为夏至新麦已经登场,古代人比较讲究"不时不食"的理念,要吃最新鲜的当季食材,所以夏至食面也有尝新的意思。冬至吃饺子是因为北方地区冬天十分寒冷,百姓的耳朵常常被冻伤,名医张仲景为了治疗人们的冻伤,用羊肉和大葱等制作饺子,人们吃了以后在寒冷的冬天能够驱寒暖胃,加速血液循环,提高身体的抗寒能力。

One should eat noodles at the summer solstice. Because ancient people prefer fresh ingredients, and the summer solstice is the time to harvest wheat, the raw material for noodles. The reason for eating dumplings at the winter solstice is because it is very cold in the northern region in winter, and people's ears are often frostbited. In order to treat people's ears, Zhang Zhongjing, a famous doctor, used mutton and green onions to make dumplings. Eating dumplings in the cold winter can help people dispel cold and warm their stomachs, accelerate blood circulation and improve their ability to resist the cold.

------ 健康小提示 -------------------------------- **Health-preserving Tips**

面汤中还含有消化酶,在煮的过程中也不会被破坏,可以帮助消化食物。

The noodle soup contains digestive enzymes, which will not be destroyed under high temperature and can help people digest food.

18　白露身不露,寒露脚不露。

One should not wear clothes with bare arms after White Dew and should keep the feet warm after Cold Dew.

白露节气一过,穿衣服就不能再赤膊露体;寒露节气一过,应注重脚部保暖。因为两脚离心脏最远,血液供应较少,再加上脚的脂肪层很薄,保温性能差,容易受凉。

One should not wear clothes with bare arms any longer after White Dew (one of the 24 solar terms). One should keep the feet warm after Cold Dew (one of the 24 solar terms). Because the feet are farthest from the heart, the blood supplied to the feet is much less, and the fat layer of the feet is very thin, which has poor thermal insulation performance, therefore the feet are easily affected by the cold weather.

----- 健康小提示 ----------------------------------- **Health-preserving Tips**

冬天最好每天用热水泡脚,水温可控制在 55~70℃。在睡前用热水泡脚,可行气活血,舒筋通络。若在泡脚的同时,再对足心足趾的穴位进行按摩,还具有消除疲劳、有助睡眠之功效。

In winter, one should soak the feet with hot water every day, and the water temperature should be controlled between 55－70℃. People can soak the feet with hot water before going to bed to promote *qi* and blood circulation and relax muscles and collaterals. One can also massage the acupoints of the feet and toes while soaking the feet, which can relieve fatigue and help sleep.

19　冬不欲极温,夏不欲穷凉。

One should not be indulged in too much heat in winter; one should not be indulged in too much coolness in summer.

"冬不欲极温,夏不欲穷凉"语出晋代葛洪的《抱朴子》。一般来说,善养生的人,顺四时而适寒温,春夏养阳,秋冬养阴。

"One should not be indulged in too much heat in winter; one should not be indulged in too much coolness in summer." The sentence comes out of *Bao Pu Zi* by Ge Hong of the Jin Dynasty. Generally speaking, people who are good at keeping healthy conform to the temperature of the four seasons, nourishing *yang* in spring and summer, while nourishing *yin* in autumn and winter.

----- **健康小提示** ---------------------------- **Health-preserving Tips**

冬天可以用凉水洗脸。夏天开空调时,室内与室外的温差不能太大,一般在5~10℃为宜。如果温差过大,人进出时经受气温骤变,容易感冒。

One can wash face with cool water in winter. When the air conditioner is turned on in summer, the difference between indoor and outdoor temperature should not be too excessive, and 5-10℃ is the most suitable temperature difference range. Otherwise, one is prone to has a cold due to the sudden change of temperature when entering and leaving the room.

20　三九补一冬,来年无病痛。

One can nourish the body in *Sanjiu* (the third nine-day period after the winter solstice) , and he/she won't get sick in the coming year.

在冬季,我们脏腑的阴阳气血会有所偏衰,合理进补能够及时补充气血,抵御严寒侵袭,还可减小来年生病概率,从而使养生效果事半功倍。

In winter, the *yin*, *yang*, *qi* and blood of our internal organs will become weak. Reasonable tonics can replenish *qi* and blood in time, resist the invasion of severe cold, and reduce the probability of illness in the coming year to achieve the goal of health maintenance more effective.

----- **健康小提示** ---------------------------- **Health-preserving Tips**

在冬季进补时最好食补、药补相结合。应本着"因人施膳"的原则,根据自身情况,选择最适合自己的补品。

One had better combine food tonic and medicine tonic in winter. Health preserving should be based on the principle of "feeding according to the person himself". One should choose the most suitable nutrition according to the physique.

21 冬季养生宜多食热粥。

One should eat more hot porridge to keep healthy in winter.

冬天可适当多摄入富含碳水化合物、脂肪及维生素的食物。粥的主要原料多为谷物类,含有一定量的蛋白质、脂肪,以及各种微量元素,有益于人体健康,因此说"冬季养生宜多食热粥"。

One should eat food rich in carbohydrates, fats and vitamins in the winter. The main raw material of porridge is the grain, which is rich in protein, fat and various trace elements. It is good for health. Therefore, there is a proverb that "One should eat more hot porridge to keep healthy in winter."

----- 健康小提示 ----------------------------- **Health-preserving Tips**

冬天感冒的人多喝热粥有助于发汗、散热、祛风寒,促进感冒的痊愈。另外,肠胃消化系统不好时,喝粥可以促进营养的吸收。

Drinking more hot porridge when one catches a cold in winter will help he/she sweat, dissipate heat, expel wind-cold, and promote the cure of colds. In addition, when one's digestive system is not good, drinking porridge can promote nutrient absorption.

22 冬令进补莫过量,合理膳食重营养。

Don't replenish the body excessively in winter, a reasonable and nutritious diet is the most important.

虽然冬季是进补的最佳时节,但是由于这个季节天气干燥,所以进补要适度,否则很有可能出现鼻腔热烘、咽喉发干、脸上冒痘痘等症状,中医认为这多是"上火"引起的。饮食均衡,保证充足的睡眠才符合养生观念。

Although it is the best time to nourish ourselves in winter, due to the dry air in this season, the tonic should be moderate, otherwise it is likely to cause hot and dry nasal cavity, dry throat, and acne on the face. TCM believes that this is mostly caused by "getting too much internal heat". A balanced diet and adequate sleep are in line with the concept of health preserving.

------ **健康小提示** ---------------------------------- **Health-preserving Tips**

冬天上火没必要立刻去药店,大白菜和白萝卜这两种冬天常见的蔬菜,便是去火的"良药"。

One doesn't need to take medicine immediately if he/she gets too much internal heat in winter. Chinese cabbage and white radish, two common vegetables in winter, are the "good medicine" to reduce internal heat.

参考书目
Works Cited

［1］黄帝内经·素问［M］.李照国,刘希茹,译.西安:世界图书出版西安公司, 2005.

［2］陶弘景. 养性延命录［M］. 北京:中国医药科技出版社, 2017.

［3］龚廷贤. 寿世保元［M］. 北京:中国中医药出版社, 1993.

［4］高红敏.《黄帝内经》中的谚语养生［M］. 北京:朝华出版社, 2009.

［5］朱熹,吕祖谦. 近思录［M］. 上海:上海古籍出版社, 2010.

［6］黄玮. 代代永流传的科学养生智慧［M］. 江西:江西科学技术出版社, 2010.

［7］张妍,刘丽娜. 老祖宗的养生经［M］. 青岛:青岛出版社, 2014.

［8］郭霞珍. 养生名言谚语集锦［M］. 北京:人民卫生出版社, 2011.

［9］丁福保. 少年进德录［M］.北京:中国发展出版社, 2003.

［10］温长路. 民谣谚语话养生［M］. 北京:中国中医药出版社, 2010.

［11］张恒. 健康百谚［M］. 北京:中国华侨出版社, 2005.

［12］温端政. 中国俗语大辞典［M］. 上海:上海辞书出版社, 2011.

［13］司马迁. 史记［M］.长沙:岳麓书社, 2019.

［14］张湖德,马烈光. 趣话中医养生经［M］. 北京:化学工业出版社, 2007.

［15］论语［M］. 许渊冲,译.北京:五洲传播出版社, 2019.

［16］钱大昕. 恒言录［M］. 上海:上海古籍出版社, 1996.

［17］蔡东藩. 前汉演义［M］. 北京:民主与建设出版社, 2020.

［18］陈君慧. 谚语大全［M］. 哈尔滨:北方文艺出版社, 2013.

［19］葛洪. 抱朴子［M］. 上海:上海古籍出版社, 1990.

［20］许沈华. 四季养生谚语［M］.2 版. 北京:人民卫生出版社, 2017.

［21］梁章钜. 退庵随笔［M］. 江苏:广陵古籍刻印社, 1997.

［22］傅昭原. 处世悬镜诠解［M］.天津:天津古籍出版社, 2018.

［23］刘仲宇,高毓秋. 中国古代养生格言［M］.上海:上海人民出版社, 2000.

［24］孟子：汉英对照［M］.赵甄陶,译.长沙：湖南人民出版社,1999.

［25］本草纲目选：汉英对照［M］.罗希文,译.北京：外文出版社,2012.

［26］刘丹彤,张小勇.养生秘旨［M］.北京：中国医药科技出版社,2017.

［27］朱彝尊.明诗综［M］.上海：上海古籍出版社,1993.

［28］张鲁原.中华古谚语大辞典［M］.上海：上海大学出版社,2011.

［29］胡文焕.类修要诀［M］.北京：中医古籍出版社,1987.

［30］孙思邈.备急千金要方［M］.北京：中国医药科技出版社,2017.

［31］徐志成.实用谚语小辞典［M］.西安：世界图书出版西安公司,2005.

［32］陆九渊.象山语录［M］.上海：上海古籍出版社,2020.

［33］赵孟頫.闲居赋·秋声赋［M］.长春：吉林文史出版社,2008.

［34］增广贤文［M］.马婷婷,译.蒙特马利：美国南方出版社,2021.

［35］王志新.汉书［M］.北京：团结出版社,2018.

［36］李梴.医学入门［M］.北京：中国中医药出版社,1995.

［37］祝总骧.祝总骧三一二经络锻炼法［M］.北京：北京体育学院出版社,2001.

［38］吴宇峰,寇馨云.寿世传真［M］.北京：中国医药科技出版社,2017.

［39］高武.针灸聚英［M］.北京：中国中医药出版社,2007.

［40］杨继洲.针灸大成［M］.天津：天津科学技术出版社,2017.

［41］*Huangdi's Canon of Medicine*［M］. Translated by Li Zhaoguo, Liu Xiru. Xi'an：World Publishing Cooperation, 2005.

［42］Tao Hongjing. *Recordings of the Healing Art for Health and Health Preservation*［M］. Beijing：China Medical Science Press, 2017.

［43］Gong Tingxian. *Shoushi Baoyuan*［M］. Beijing：China Press of Traditional Chinese Medicine, 1993.

［44］Gao Hongmin. *Proverbs about Health Preservation in "Huangdi Neijing"*［M］. Beijing：Blossom Press, 2009.

［45］Zhu Xi, Lü Zuqian. *Reflections on Things at Hand*［M］. Shanghai：Shanghai Classics Publishing House, 2010.

［46］Huang Wei. *The Scientific Health Preservation passed down from Generation to Generation*［M］. Jiangxi：Jiangxi Science and Technology Press, 2010.

［47］Zhang Yan, Liu Lina. *Health Preservation Classic Left by Ancestors*［M］. Qingdao：Qingdao Publishing House, 2014.

［48］Guo Xiazhen. *Collection of Well-known Sayings and Proverbs about Health Preservation*［M］. Beijing：People's Medical Publishing House, 2011.

［49］Ding Fubao. *Records of Cultivating Virtues*［M］. Beijing：China Development

Press，2003.

［50］Wen Changlu. *Health Preservation in Folk Proverbs*［M］. Beijing：China Press of Traditional Chinese Medicine，2010.

［51］Zhang Heng. *A hundred Proverbs of Health*［M］. Beijing：The Chinese Overseas Publishing House，2005.

［52］Wen Duanzheng. *Dictionary of Ancient Chinese Proverbs*［M］. Shanghai：Shanghai Lexi-
cographical Publishing House，2011.

［53］Sima Qian. *Records of the Grand Historian*［M］. Changsha：Yuelu Press，2019.

［54］Zhang Hude, Ma Lieguang. *Witty Remark on Health Preservation Classic of Traditional
Chinese Medicine*［M］. Beijing：Chemical Industry Press，2007.

［55］*The Analects*［M］. Translated by Xu Yuanchong. Beijing：Intercontinental Communication
Center，2019.

［56］Qian Daxin. *Records of Common Saying*［M］. Shanghai：Shanghai Classics Publishing
House，1996.

［57］Cai Dongfan. *Romance in the Early Han Dynasty*［M］. Beijing：Democracy & Construction
Press，2020.

［58］Chen Junhui. *Proverbs*［M］. Harbin：The North Literature and Art Publishing House，
2013.

［59］Ge Hong. *The Master Who Embraces Simplicity*［M］. Shanghai：Shanghai Classics Publishing House，1990.

［60］Xu Shenhua. *Proverbs about Health Preservation in Four Seasons*［M］. 2nd ed. Beijing：
People's Medical Publishing House，2017.

［61］Liang Zhangju. *Essay of Tui Yan*［M］. Jiangsu：Guangling Classics Engraving Agency，
1997.

［62］Fu Zhaoyuan. *Interpretation of Wisdom of Conducting Yourself*［M］. Tianjin：Tianjin
Classics Publishing House，2018.

［63］Liu Zhongyu, Gao Yuqiu. *Chinese Ancient Health Preservation Motto*［M］. Shanghai：
Shanghai People's Publishing House，2000.

［64］*Chinese-English Contrast of Mencius*［M］. Translated by Zhao Zhentao. Changsha：Hunan
People's Publishing House，1999.

［65］*Chinese-English Contrast of Compendium of Materia Medica*［M］. Translated by Luo Xi-
wen. Beijing：Foreign Languages Press，2012.

［66］Liu Dantong, Zhang Xiaoyong. *Secret Documents of Health Preservation*［M］. Beijing：
China Medical Science Press，2017.

[67] Zhu Yizun. *A Collection of Poem in the Ming Dynasty*[M]. Shanghai：Shanghai Classics Publishing House, 1993.

[68] Zhang Luyuan. *Dictionary of Ancient Chinese Proverbs*[M]. Shanghai：Shanghai University Press, 2011.

[69] Hu Wenhuan. *Key to Preserving Health* [M]. Beijing：Classics of Traditional Chinese Medicine Publishing House, 1987.

[70] Sun Simiao. *Golden Prescriptions for Emergency Use*[M]. Beijing：China Medical Science Press, 2017.

[71] Xu Zhicheng. *Dictionary of Practical Proverbs*[M]. Xi'an：World Publishing Cooperation, 2005.

[72] Lu Jiuyuan. *Important words Spoken in Xiang Mountain*[M]. Shanghai：Shanghai Classics Publishing House, 2020.

[73] Zhao Mengfu. *Odes to the Sound of Autumn & Living in Idleness* [M]. Changchun：Jilin Literature and History Publishing House, 2008.

[74] Wang Zhixin. *Book of Han*[M]. Beijing：Unity Press, 2018.

[75] Li Ting. *Introduction to Medicine*[M]. Beijing：China Press of Traditional Chinese Medicine, 1995.

[76] Zhu Zongxiang. *Zhu Zongxiang's* 312 *Meridians Exercise Method*[M]. Beijing：Beijing Institute of Physical Education Press, 2001.

[77] Wu Yufeng, Kou Xinyun. *A Book of Longevity* [M]. Beijing：China Medical Science Press, 2017.

[78] Gao Wu. *A Book of Acupuncture and Moxibustion*[M]. Beijing：China Press of Traditional Chinese Medicine, 2007.

[79] Yang Jizhou. *Complete Works of Acupuncture and Moxibustion*[M]. Tianjin：Tianjin Science and Technology Press, 2017.

附 录
APPENDICES

附录1　中医术语汉英对照表

中文	英文
精神	essence and spirit
虚实	deficiency and excess
七情	seven emotions
喜	joy
怒	rage
忧	worry
思	pensiveness
悲	grief
恐	terror
惊	fright
五脏六腑	five *zang* viscera and six *fu* viscera
气功	*qigong*
太极拳	*taijiquan*
八段锦	*baduanjin*（eight-sectioned exercise）
气机	*qi* movement
心神	heart spirit

（续表）

中文	英文
心	heart
肝	liver
脾	spleen
肺	lung
肾	kidney
情志	emotion
天人合一	harmony between man and nature
疏肝理气	soothe the liver and regulate *qi*
取象比类	classification according to manifestation
肝火	liver fire
气血不畅/失调	disharmony of *qi* and blood
气血不足	insufficiency of *qi* and blood
经络	meridian
宽胸理气	soothe the chest and regulate *qi*
阴气	*yin qi*
阳气	*yang qi*
阴阳不和	disharmony of *yin* and *yang*
五志	five minds
气逆	*qi* counterflow
气血紊乱	disorders of *qi* and blood
气血运行	circulation of *qi* and blood
五体	five body constituents
郁气	stagnant *qi*
正气	healthy *qi*
元气	original *qi*
性凉	cool in nature

（续表）

中文	英文
消食	promote digestion
解毒	detoxify
补虚	tonify deficiency
健脾开胃	invigorate the spleen and increase the appetite
强肾阴	strengthen the kidney *yin*
温补阳气	warm and tonify *yang qi*
滋补脾胃	nourish the stomach and spleen
阴虚阳亢	*yin* deficiency and *yang* hyperactivity
胃气	stomach *qi*
温中止痛	warm the middle and relieve pain
行气	promote *qi*
湿邪	dampness pathogen
益气	replenish *qi*
生津润燥	promote body fluid and moisten dryness
清热解毒	clear heat and relieve toxin
发汗解表	induce sweating to release the exterior
清热除烦	clear heat and eliminate irritability
平肝调经	pacify liver and regulate menstruation
凉血消肿	cool blood to alleviate edema
疏通气血	free the *qi* and blood
散风清热	disperse wind and clear heat
清肝明目	clear liver and improve vision
解毒消炎	remove toxin to eliminate inflammation
滋阴补阳	nourish *yin* and *yang*
补中益气	tonify middle and replenish *qi*
养血安神	nourish blood and induce tranquilization

（续表）

中文	英文
补肾固精	tonify kidney and secure essence
润肺定喘	moisten lung to arrest panting
润肠通便	moisten intestines to relieve constipation
健胃补血	invigorate stomach and tonify blood
惊悸	fright palpitation
活血散瘀	activate blood to dissipate stasis
清热解暑	clear the heat and release the summerheat
生津	engender fluid
健胃消食	invigorate the stomach and promote digestion
健脾温中	invigorate the spleen and warm the middle
消炎利尿	eliminate inflammation to promote urination
消瘀凉血	dissipate stasis and cool blood
顺气镇咳	smooth *qi* and settle cough
消暑生津	clear summer heat and engender fluid
阴虚	*yin* deficiency
补气生血	replenish *qi* and produce blood
解表散寒	release the exterior and disperse cold
温中止呕	warm the middle and stop vomiting
温肺止咳	warm lung and stop cough
调经止痛	regulate menstruation to relieve pain
润燥滑肠	moisten dryness to smooth the intestines
驱寒发汗	dispel cold and induce sweat
祛湿利尿	remove dampness and promote urination
舌质	tongue body
舌苔	tongue coating
小便不利	inhibited urination

（续表）

中文	英文
消炎降火	eliminate inflammation to reduce fire
理气化痰	regulate *qi* and resolve phlegm
散结	dissipate nodulation
五味	five flavors
酸苦甘辛咸	sour, bitter, sweet, pungent and salty
痰浊	phlegm turbidity
肝气郁结	stagnation of liver *qi*
热毒	heat toxin
三焦	triple energizer
胃气	stomach *qi*
脏腑	*zang-fu* organs
滋阴凉血	nourish *yin* and cool blood
滋阴生津	nourish *yin* to engender fluid
清热利湿	clear heat and drain damp
便溏	loose stool
润肺止咳	moisten lung and stop cough
养心安神	nourish heart and induce tranquilization
健脾和胃	invigorate spleen and harmonize stomach
暑湿之邪	summer-damp pathogen
风邪	wind pathogen

附录 2　穴位汉英对照表

中文	英文
阴陵泉	*Yinlingquan*（SP 9）
足三里穴	*Zusanli*（ST 36）
涌泉穴	*Yongquan*（KI 1）
劳宫穴	*Laogong*（PC 8）
昆仑穴	*Kunlun*（BL 60）
委中穴	*Weizhong*（BL 40）
承山穴	*Chengshan*（BL 57）
列缺穴	*Lieque*（LU 7）
太冲穴	*Taichong*（LR 3）
足太阴脾经	the spleen meridian of foot taiyin（SP）
足少阴肾经	the kidney meridian of foot shaoyin（KI）

附录3　常用中药汉英对照表

中文	拼音	英文	拉丁文
黄芪	*huangqi*	milkvetch root	*Radix Astragali seu Hedysari*
当归	*danggui*	Chinese angelica	*Radix Angelicae Sinensis*
生姜	*shengjiang*	fresh ginger	*Rhizoma Zingiberis Recens*
山药	*shanyao*	common yam rhizome	*Rhizoma Dioscoreae*
丁香	*dingxiang*	clove	*Flos Caryophylli*
茴香	*huixiang*	fennel	*Fructus Foeniculi*
胡椒	*hujiao*	pepper fruit	*Fructus Piperis Nigri*
马齿苋	*machixian*	purslane herb	*Herba Portulacae*
白术	*baizhu*	largehead atractylodes rhizome	*Rhizoma Atractylodis Macrocephalae*
阿胶	*ejiao*	ass hide glue	*Colla Corii Asini*
艾叶	*aiye*	argy wormwood leaf	*Folium Artemisiae Argyi*
茯苓	*fuling*	Indian bread	*Poria*
石斛	*shihu*	dendrobium	*Herba Dendrobii*
百合	*baihe*	lily	*Bulbus Lilii*
灵芝	*lingzhi*	glossy ganoderma	*Ganoderma*

附录4　中医典籍汉英对照表

中文	拼音	英文
《防病贵早》	Fang Bing Gui Zao	Preventing Disease in Advance
《黄帝内经》	Huang Di Nei Jing	Huangdi's Canon of Medicine
《恒言录》	Heng Yan Lu	Records of Common Saying
《前汉演义》	Qian Han Yan Yi	The Romance in the Early Han Dynasty
《抱朴子》	Bao Pu Zi	The Master Who Embraces Simplicity
《产经》	Chan Jing	Records of Gynaecological and Paediatric Diseases
《退庵随笔》	Tui Yan Sui Bi	Essay of Tui Yan
《处世悬镜》	Chu Shi Xuan Jing	Wisdom of Conducting Yourself
《神农本草经》	Shen Nong Ben Cao Jing	Shennong's Classic of Medicinal Herbs
《河东谚》	He Dong Yan	Proverbs in the East of the Yellow River
《养生要集》	Yang Sheng Yao Ji	A Collection of Health Preservation
《本草纲目》	Ben Cao Gang Mu	Compendium of Materia Medica
《备急千金要方》	Bei Ji Qian Jin Yao Fang	Golden Prescriptions for Emergency Use
《养生秘旨》	Yang Sheng Mi Zhi	Secret Documents of Health Preservation
《明诗综》	Ming Shi Zong	A Collection of Poem in the Ming Dynasty
《类修要诀》	Lei Xiu Yao Jue	Key to Preserving Health
《象山语录》	Xiang Shan Yu Lu	Important Words Spoken in Xiang Mountain
《闲居赋·秋声赋》	Xian Ju Fu · Qiu Sheng Fu	Odes to the Sound of Autumn & Living in Idleness
《增广贤文》	Zeng Guang Xian Wen	The Wisdom of Ancient Aphorisms
《汉书》	Han Shu	Book of Han
《医学入门》	Yi Xue Ru Men	Introduction to Medicine
《寿世传真》	Shou Shi Chuan Zhen	A Book of Longevity
《针灸聚英》	Zhen Jiu Ju Yiing	A Book of Acupuncture and Moxibustion
《针灸大成》	Zhen Jiu Da Cheng	Complete Works of Acupuncture and Moxibustion
《养性延命录》	Yang Xing Yan Ming Lu	A Collection of Health Preservation